Christoph Ribbat
Breathing in Manhattan

Culture & Theory | Volume 287

Christoph Ribbat is a Professor of American Studies at Universität Paderborn (Germany). He was a Humboldt Fellow at MIT and Boston University and a Fulbright Scholar at The Cooper Union, New York. His work has been translated into fourteen languages.

Christoph Ribbat
Breathing in Manhattan
Carola Speads – The German Jewish Gymnastics
Instructor Who Brought Mindfulness to America

[transcript]

Bibliographic information published by the Deutsche Nationalbibliothek
The Deutsche Nationalbibliothek lists this publication in the Deutsche Nationalbibliografie; detailed bibliographic data are available in the Internet at http://dnb.d-nb.de

© 2023 transcript Verlag, Bielefeld

All rights reserved. No part of this book may be reprinted or reproduced or utilized in any form or by any electronic, mechanical, or other means, now known or hereafter invented, including photocopying and recording, or in any information storage or retrieval system, without permission in writing from the publisher.

Cover layout: Maria Arndt, Bielefeld
Cover illustration: Carola Speads' New York studio, detail (unknown photographer, from the Papers of Carola and Otto Spitz)
Printed by: Majuskel Medienproduktion GmbH, Wetzlar
https://doi.org/10.14361/9783839467091
Print-ISBN 978-3-8376-6709-7
PDF-ISBN 978-3-8394-6709-1
ISSN of series: 2702-8968
eISSN of series: 2702-8976

Printed on permanent acid-free text paper.

Contents

1. The Studio of Physical Re-Education 7
2. Wandervögel 27
3. Notice What Is 43
4. The List of Jewish Gymnastics Instructors 61
5. Flowers from Charlotte 83
6. Speads Work 97
Sources 113
Illustrations 117
Notes 119

1. The Studio of Physical Re-Education

The relaxation expert isn't relaxed. Her neck hurts. She's looking out the window, to the East. She gazes at the trees, the meadows, the lake. The rent for this apartment is way too high. She can't stop thinking about that. And then again, what a treat it is to see so much of this vast sky, the sun and the clouds and seagulls soaring.

Her marriage isn't working very well. Otto's so desperate. And the split from Charlotte is eating her up inside. She, Carola, once called her Charlöttchen, and Charlöttchen called her Carölchen. They worked together for more than ten years. They were like sisters. Together they went through extremely hard times. Now they don't speak anymore. And Frau Gindler, who really should be on Carola's side, refuses to comment. What Frau Gindler thinks is very important to Carola.

She observes how the wind makes streaks on the surface of the water and how these patterns change constantly. She looks at the trees and the narrow paths that weave their way through the green. Behind the trees she sees the Metropolitan Museum on Fifth Avenue. Behind the museum there's the Upper East Side and the East River and Queens and Long Island and then the Atlantic and then Europe. She regularly takes the bus to Germany.

Her clients will be arriving soon. The straws are ready. She doesn't use the big ones meant for milkshakes, but the small ones used for cocktails. The straw experiment is one of her trademarks. She hears the distant sounds of the cars ten floors below her. This light, empty room up here is her workplace: She has named it the "Studio of Physical Re-Education."

She is 53 years old. Legally, her name is Carola Henrietta Spitz. To her clients, she's Carola Speads. In an old passport she was Carola Spitzová and, before that, Carola Joseph. She was called Molle for a while during her childhood, at a point when she was a little chubby, "mollig" in German. Her mother continued to call her Molle even as an adult, even when she wrote her last letter from Amsterdam.

It's autumn, 1954. Sometimes she takes the bus that crosses the park at 86th Street. Then it's just a few more blocks and she's in Yorkville. "Little Germany." Schaller & Weber on Second Avenue stock German apple sauce, pickles and Pumpernickel, as well as Leberwurst and "German Blockwurst."[1] The pork doesn't bother her. Her husband's a Jew. She's a Jew. They also have a Christmas tree every year, just as they had back in Berlin.

The expensive building she's been living in for almost a year is called Rossleigh Court. It sits on the corner of 85th Street and Central Park West. This means she has two addresses. For her private mail she uses 1 West 85th Street. She gets a lot of letters to that address, many from German authorities and a lawyer in West Berlin. Herr Schwarz is a reparations specialist. He himself lost his father in the Theresienstadt camp.[2] She exchanges complicated and painful things with him.

As her professional address, for the Studio of Physical Re-Education, she uses 251 Central Park West. Everyone in New York knows what that means. What a fantastic location that is. What the view must be like. Rossleigh Court may not rank as the most glamourous building in the city, but the luxurious towers of the Eldorado loom just a few blocks to the left. And down to the right: the Dakota.

When you cross the street here, you walk into another world, the green park, where the air, filtered by the trees, feels incredibly fresh. In 1950s New York, hundreds of thousands of coal heaters, thousands of incinerators, and countless busses, trucks, and cars are giving off smoke. Masses of commuters are driving their automobiles over newly built highways from the suburbs into the city. That is a very modern concept of the way people should live. You see soot everywhere. Some days you'd think the New York air consisted only of exhaust.³ Here by the park, of course, things are different.

It's a quiet building. The walls are thick. You don't notice the neighbors much. Rumor has it that the Croatian family on the eighth floor had relationships with the SS and therefore welcomed the prospect of a postwar escape to New York. On the eleventh floor lives Alberta Szalita. During the war she worked as a neurologist in a Moscow hospital. There, in the autumn of 1943, Szalita received a message that her husband, her father, her mother, four of her sisters, and one of her grandfathers had been killed in a German-organized mass shooting. Szalita emigrated to the United States. She trained as a psychoanalyst. She tried to come to terms with her relationships to the murdered, as impossible as that seemed. She'd run away from mourning, Szalita later writes, and mourning caught up with her.⁴

That is a fate shared by many on the Upper West Side. But most stay silent on issues like these. Many still run away. Carola could tell stories about the unimaginable suffering of her mother and brother, or of her own experiences in Berlin, Amsterdam, and Paris. She doesn't, though. She doesn't even tell Stevie, Alan, and Johnny. Later, as successful men in their sixties, her grandsons will say that their "Omi" hadn't wanted to compromise their American lives. They come over regularly, the little boys, often on Saturday afternoons when Carola's weekend classes are over. Sometimes they stay the night. Omi tells them about the dog she had as a little girl and who was allowed to sleep in bed with her, in Berlin, back in the day. A German shepherd.

This summer, in June, sirens wailed here in New York. The city pretended it was going to be struck by atomic bombs. Operation Alert took place one Monday. Three H-bombs fell on the city. That was the scenario. One hit Queens, one the Bronx, and one Manhattan, right at First Avenue and 57th Street. New Yorkers vacated the sidewalks and headed for the designated shelters. The drill was supposed to strengthen their belief that their country could deal with anything, even the most monstrous attack. Realists say, however, that these three bombs would have killed more than two million people and that the designated shelters wouldn't have helped much.⁵

Her clients in the Studio of Physical Re-Education are seeking another kind of protection. Carola's empty room up here is a place where they feel safe. Some get out of the subway at 86th Street. They leave the rumbling, the creaking, and the darkness behind them. They climb the stairs into the daylight, walk alongside the building and turn right on 85th Street. The entrance is right there. In the lobby a sign says: ALL VISITORS & DELIVERIES MUST BE ANNOUNCED: PLEASE COOPERATE WITH THE DOORMAN. A while later another sign will say: THIS IS A SMOKE-FREE BUILDING. The clients cooperate with the doorman.

She has a client, an anthropologist, who coined the term "culture shock." Cora Du Bois did fieldwork on the island of Alor, Indonesia, alone in what for her was a completely alien world. Du Bois observed that the first two months in another culture seem like completely lost time. First you have to process the shock of the foreign, become accustomed to the manners, the unfamiliar food, the body language. Du Bois wants to find out whether there's any way to adapt more quickly, react more flexibly to change. Carola's teachings seem to prepare for exactly that.⁶

Personally, though, Carola has had different experiences. She's lived here for fourteen years. She's been an American citizen since March 1946. And for some reason, she can't get past her own "culture shock."

At the beginning she couldn't face the subway. Employees were stationed on the platforms, shoving people into the jammed cars, their backsides, shoulders, heads. Back then she lived in Washington Heights in northern Manhattan, and she worked in Midtown. She got on at 191st Street, almost at the beginning of the line, and even then she had to squash herself into an already crammed car. On her journey home from 57th Street, things were far worse.

Now other things horrify her. She notes the "impossible struggle for survival" in America and the excesses of capitalism. The way people live only "for their own personal gain." She says it's "simply indescribable." She's surprised when people here simply behave "properly" for once. In the papers, she reads about kids who beat their parents to death, about parents who murder their own children, and about contract killings, carried out for a couple of dollars. That's the American way of life.

Fig. 1: Carola Spitz, 1946.

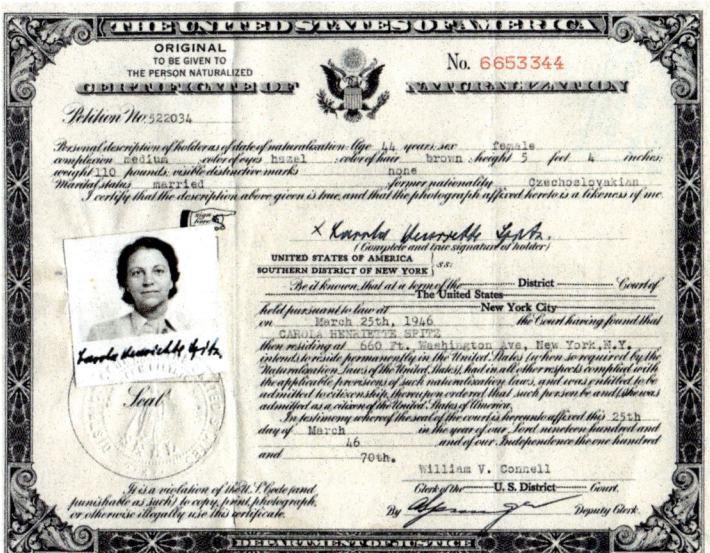

Anybody who is scared, says the expert Carola Speads, will have a changed body. It's a natural process. The body wants to help you overcome the emergency that fear creates. But what happens when the fear remains? Then alertness changes into something else. Your body tenses up. The muscles stay strained, the joints stiff, the breathing shallow. The tension can lead to an overwhelming struggle that could result in complete flaccidness. It's a vicious cycle, Speads says. Because a fearful person can't properly command their muscles, tendons, or breath, they adopt other postures, meaning that the tension or the flaccidness will spread further, and the person will become even more fearful.

What helps? Breathing. 24 years from now, in 1978 – she'll still be living in this apartment – she will publish a book about the subject. She'll state that the modern individual lives in a breathless time. And in her book that's not a figurative expression. She will shine a light on the difference between disrupted breath and satisfactory breath and demonstrate that all aspects of life are influenced by breathing. Those who master the art of satisfactory breathing, Speads' study says, will also get a handle on the larger things in life.[7]

Carola's career began in 1920s Berlin. Everyone in her circles there knew "the Kofler," his *Art of Breathing*, the standard work. There was no getting around Kofler. He recommended the "invigorating effect" of the "lung sweeper" (breathe in through a tiny opening in the lips), the sip exercise, the muscle exercise for the crescendo and decrescendo, plus the exercise improving elasticity. Not to forget the guiding principle: "take breaths through the nose."[8] For Carola, however, Kofler's exercises have never been enough. She doesn't want to just guide singers to better singing or actors to a sturdier voice. She rejects the notion that one can breathe better or worse or rightly or wrongly. Her studio is a place of research. She wants to investigate breath and the body. Like Elsa Gindler, back in Berlin. In her studio in Kurfürstenstraße, Gindler hadn't focused on exercises, repetition, and corrections, but on the mindful exploration of one's own body. She'd had answers to Carola's questions and Carola later exported Gindler's ideas to New York.

Down in the lobby of her building, her clients walk past the mailboxes and toward one of the elevators that will take them up to mindfulness. There are six elevators in Rossleigh Court: two for the service staff, four for more distinguished passengers. Once the clients have arrived, high up in the building, they enter the apartment, turn left, and walk into one of the dressing rooms. These two small compartments remind some clients poignantly of high school. They take some things off and put relatively few things back on. The women enter the studio in bathing suits. The men are wearing swimming trunks. Carola sits on the windowsill. She's ready to breathe with them.

Everyone breathes, but who really thinks about breathing? Poets maybe, because every line of a poem is limited to the length of a breath. Elizabeth Bishop, a postwar poet nine years younger than Carola, composes an ode named "O Breath." In the poem someone watches a naked woman breathing. That someone observes how the little hairs on the nipples of her lover move. One breast has four hairs, the other five. It's a complicated poem about the desire to know more about the other, about not being able to look inside them, and about watching only this movement: the fluttering of these hairs. "O Breath" does not flow. It falters. The asthmatic Elizabeth Bishop concentrates on the difficulties of breathing. She shows how words and ideas form when the breath comes irregularly, painfully, heavily.[9] Maybe the only people who think about breathing are those who have difficulty doing so. Everyone else takes it for granted.

After her arrival in New York in 1940, Carola quickly teamed up with Charlotte. She'd already been friends with her in Germany. They had a lot in common: they'd both been gymnastics instructors, were both born in 1901, and both came from well-off families. They'd also both lost almost everything when they emigrated. Because the Gindler method was virtually unknown in the United States, Charlotte and Carola tried this niche to maybe earn a living. They rented a tiny studio near Carnegie Hall. Pronounced in an American accent, Carola's name sounded like "Carola spits." That had to be changed. Then Speads and Selver began to promote their gymnastics.

In the early 1940s, 70,000 German refugees set out to do exactly what Carola and Charlotte were doing: to somehow survive in New York City. Social decline was the norm. Among refugees there was a popular joke about a dachshund who said to another dachshund that, back in Europe, he'd been a St. Bernhard.[10] Older people had a particularly hard time. That was the case for Carola's neighbors in Washington Heights, the Kissingers. The father, heavily depressed, never got used to life in America. As a result, his wife had to work as a cook, and his son Heinz, later Henry, a classmate of Carola's daughter, worked in a shaving brush factory. It was impossible to say what could become of a refugee boy like Heinz/Henry Kissinger, with his heavy German accent.

Carola and Charlotte had their German degrees as gymnastics instructors. These diplomas were worth a lot to them and meant almost nothing here. The obstacles Speads and Selver had to face were enormous. Who wanted a German expert to improve their body when German refugees, to Americans, seemed so physically strange? There was their heavy, rigid gait. That serious, worried, almost paranoid expression. People called it "the German look." New Yorkers, far more laid-back, weren't always aware that these somber Germans had lost everything, that their closest family members had not made it out of Europe, and that they were tormented first by rumors and then by increasingly accurate news of mass executions. They saw how stiffly the Germans, in their absurd, ancient coats, took off their hats with a sweeping gesture when saying hello, and how they always bowed in this city where no one ever bowed, or, worse still, clicked their heels together. The Germans couldn't do small talk, didn't have a clue about baseball, but they still assumed they knew everything about the world. They insisted on shaking hands to say goodbye and just couldn't see how awkward that was.[11]

So Speads and Selver were two Germans planning to teach Americans how to relax. But they had no choice and so they adopted the style of New Yorkers. They had a brochure printed that set out their most important selling points in capital letters. They boasted that "THIS WORK HAS BEEN TESTED OVER MANY YEARS OF TEACHING AT UNIVERSITIES, HOSPITALS AND ART SCHOOLS." That it had been developed "IN COLLABORATION WITH MOST DISTINGUISHED SPECIALISTS." They presented Frau Gindler's mindfulness approach as a "NEW METHOD" and summarized her teachings under the heading: "THE RESULTS ARE." They knew all too well that Gindler's work wasn't a "method," that it was almost impossible to summarize, and that it hardly ever yielded simple results. They promised their prospective American clients vitality and flexibility. They looked up doctors, psychoanalysts, and orthopedists, leaving brochures in their waiting rooms, hoping for success. But the market for people with flexibility issues wasn't particularly dynamic at the time.

Now things aren't going too well between Carola and her husband. Otto works as a traveling salesman, selling on commission. He earns next to nothing. In all honesty, he's unemployed. And Otto has no idea what else to do. He's 67 years old.

Carola's studio isn't much of a success either. But Otto's American business concept really went down the drain. Soon after arriving in New York, he'd founded a women's clothing store with his brother Friedrich. Fritz to Germans, Fred to Americans. They wanted to turn both their names into the name of the store, so they settled on "Fredo." The store could be found in the heart of the Schmattes District, the fashion center of Manhattan. It went bankrupt in 1952.

In the 1950s it is spectacularly embarrassing for a family to be kept afloat by a working woman. For German refugees, other standards might apply. In the Kissinger household, for instance, the father also doesn't work. But any other couple would at least use the biggest, prettiest room of the apartment as their living room. In the Spitz residence, that space contains the Studio of Physical Re-Education. The small, dark dining room is their salon. And the question remains whether they'll be able to hold on to the apartment at all. That is Carola's most painful predicament. The students come because her studio is so beautiful. But unless more students show up soon, the beautiful studio won't be hers anymore.

And Otto is so clingy. He can't be alone; he needs her, as a partner, a friend, a listener. His brother spends a lot of time at Eclair on 72nd Street, where Central European waiters call each other "Herr Doktor," maybe because they really hold extremely high degrees, and maybe just because it sounds good. Isaac Bashevis Singer is a regular at Eclair. He always orders the tuna sandwich. He's the greatest writer in the Yiddish language.[12] And Fritz/Fred Spitz is practically just as well-known as I.B. Singer, at least at Eclair. Unlike his brother, he has a life. He's trying to start another business, another women's clothing shop. In depressing contrast, anxious Otto doesn't seem to have any plans at all.

A red enamel ashtray is sitting in one of the changing rooms on the tenth floor of 251 Central Park West. It's a wonderful object. One of Carola's clients really loves it. For years she takes part in her courses, looks at the ashtray, time and again, and one day steals it.

It isn't all that strange in those days to see an ashtray in a space devoted to mindful breathing. Of course people stub out cigarettes right before the class begins: In the early 1950s the average American smokes 3,500 cigarettes per year. Scientists are only beginning to see connections between tobacco use and lung cancer. And the war has made smoking even more popular. There's something modern, something heroic, about holding that glowing thing, and about breathing in, breathing out, and controlling stress by smoking. The cigarette can do everything. That's what the ads say.[13]

Strangely enough, though, some people want to quit smoking regardless. To them Carola recommends working with a straw or a cigarette-free cigarette holder. You breathe out through the nose, pause, then breathe in through the nose. Pause again. Put the straw or the cigarette holder in your mouth, breathe out through that little opening, gently, softly, and then, before you finish exhaling, you take out the straw or cigarette holder and breathe the rest of the air out through your nose. Gently, again. You repeat the process, and you're going to breathe out more air than you're used to and therefore also breathe in more air, and because all that oxygen will satisfy you, you won't ever want to smoke again.

The women in the bathing suits and the men in the swimming trunks are sitting on the hardwood floor. Bookshelves tower behind them. Light streams through the windows on the right. The instructor is sitting cross-legged in front of them. It just takes a few moments for everyone to quiet down. Her students see something patient and ethereal in Carola. To some of them it's her charisma alone that keeps frantic city life out of this room.

1. The Studio of Physical Re-Education   17

Fig. 2: In the Studio of Physical Re-Education (Photographer: Carola Speads).

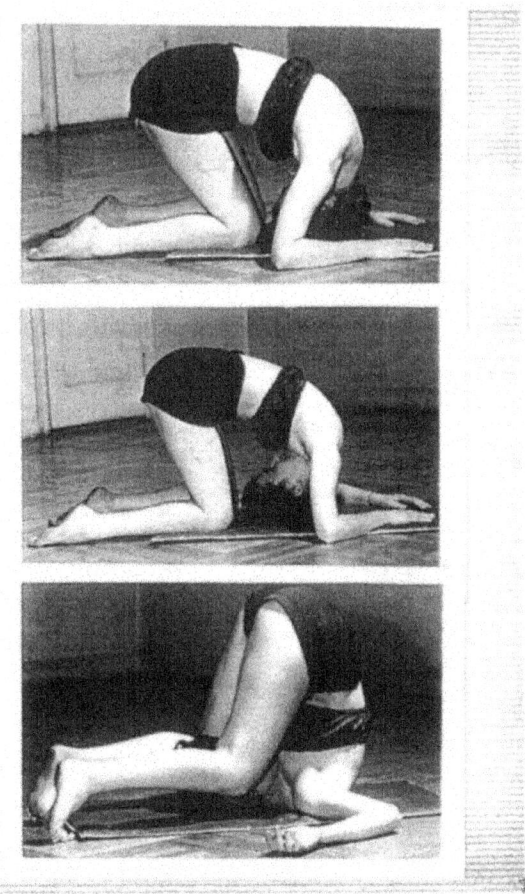

Into the silence she asks how it's going. Is anything causing problems? Does anything feel different than last week? Better? Worse? Some students speak up. Backs hurt. Heads ache. A knee has issues. But there are also those who aren't suffering from anything. They only show up because they want to learn more about themselves. These are Carola's favorite students. They have managed to understand the most important point: The more you know about your body, the better you're going to feel.

The first years in New York were tough for Carola, but they were even tougher for Charlotte. Carola at least had Otto during these hard times, a businessman with a certain degree of potential, and they had their daughter Dorothea, who did sewing piecework to contribute to the family income. All Charlotte had was an ex-husband who made her want to kill herself. In Germany Charlotte had always had servants, like Carola. In New York she became a servant herself. She worked for the enormously rich. She cleaned out their chamber pots. She acquired a masseuse's diploma to attract more high society customers. That worked out. One Mrs. Schinasi hired her. Charlotte slept in the same room as Mrs. Schinasi because when Mrs. Schinasi woke up in the middle of the night, she was only able to fall asleep again if someone massaged her millionaire heiress's feet. Stressed-out Charlotte got sick, again and again, she couldn't teach her hours in the studio, which meant that Carola had to take care not just of Charlotte, but also of Charlotte's clients.

And then one of them, just one of them, got all this attention from Martha Parker, the *New York Times* beauty columnist. During the war Parker recommended a range of innovations to her readers: the two-minute perm, for instance, and dust-repelling make-up for women working in weapon factories. Parker also solved the complex problem as to whether lipstick should be applied before powder, the method advised by Elizabeth Arden, or after powder, following Helena Rubinstein's principle (Parker developed a synthesis: lipstick and powder should be applied multiple times and intermittently.) And in December 1944 the *Times* beauty expert devoted an entire column to a form of bodywork that a certain Carola Speads had brought to town.

Speads, Parker wrote, let her students find out for themselves what was good for them. Bow down, Speads would say. Try to touch your toes and try not to bend your knees. And if that doesn't work, if you can't reach your toes, stop down there, and ask yourself: what's stopping me? Remain in that position. Just stay there, somewhere in the vicinity of knees and toes – for as long as it takes for you to know what's keeping you from doing what you wanted to do. There was nothing about Charlotte in that *New York Times* piece.[14]

After the war, Charlotte accused Carola of concentrating too much on her family: on Otto, on Dorothea. They discussed a very difficult question: Which one of them took mindfulness work more seriously? If she hadn't stepped in, of this Charlotte was certain, Carola would never have stuck to "the work." Wasn't it true that, in those early New York years, Otto had wanted Carola to work as a seamstress for him, Fritz, and Fredo, and to sew fur into ladies' coats instead of teaching mindfulness? And wasn't it Charlotte, though unrecognized by the *New York Times*, who had saved Carola from this existence as a Schmattes District sweatshop worker? Wasn't it Charlotte who had convinced her that, with all her knowledge and experience, she should never live that kind of life? Discussing these questions, the two women, once as close as sisters, grew apart.

Now, in 1954, Carola is watching the group. When she thinks that people need to move around, she asks them to close their eyes and walk on the spot. After a few minutes she proposes that they stand still. See what their breath is doing. How has it changed between standing and walking and standing again? You find out by becoming very quiet and feeling what's going on inside you. After a while you might want to move your legs again. Then stand still. Inhale. Exhale. Keep asking: What has changed?

She tells the group to walk around, eyes closed. They're in a relatively empty room. It's a large living room by New York standards. But it's still just a living room, so her clients bump into each other as they're walking around. All these people are New Yorkers, who in their everyday lives do everything they can to avoid bodily contact with random strangers. As hard as that is: by now New York City has eight million inhabitants. Add to these the three million commuters. So every workday a metropolis floods into a metropolis. Everyone seems to be on their way to work at the same time. And everyone seems to finish work at the same time. Subways, busses, sidewalks are full of people. Then the apartment you return to at night, if you're one of the eight million and not one of the commuting millions, will probably seem too small and your neighbors too close and too noisy.[15] And now, in this otherwise peaceful studio, New Yorkers are voluntarily bumping into each other, and they're scantily clad, too. Skin touches skin. It's alright to get nervous and laugh. Carola doesn't stop this. She wants her clients to notice what's going on.

The group sits back down. How has their breathing changed? How do specific body parts feel now? Carola lets them sit still for a while. She lets them report back. She listens. She lets them ask questions. She answers. Someone feels a little hot. Someone got a little scared. Someone feels tense in the shoulders. She asks about the details. She asks what it's like to perform a certain movement. People respond. Or they think in silence. She says: Good. Keep working. When someone talks too much, which happens, she states that this isn't a discussion circle. It's about feeling.

Walking the streets of Manhattan in the early 1950s, she realizes that ever so many people here seem in desperate need of Physical Re-Education. She looks at tense faces. She sees stony stares, wrinkles between eyes, chins jutted forward. She notes that people hold their breath much too often, or that they breathe too shallowly, all because they're so stressed. They're always in a hurry, so they're always out of breath. Because they're chronically stressed, their breathing issues are also chronic. Carola notes the deranged body posture when people descend stairways. How they hold on to the handrail, almost panicking for fear of falling. How they need to turn their entire body to make one foot reach the next step down. She notes how scared some people seem just because they're going to have to get off the bus.

When she gives lectures on these issues, she shows pictures of children moving around. How they frolic without fear, without inhibition, keeping their bodies straight. Our childhood is over, Carola Speads says, but we can get there again. We can re-educate ourselves and find a way back to these fluid movements. Everyone can do it: factory workers, artists, businesspeople, dancers, doctors, teachers, students, grandmothers. If you're a saleswoman, you can learn how to stand in a shop, relaxed and painless, on your feet for hours. It is also possible to type all day long, as a secretary, without tensing up in the shoulders. If you're a pianist, you can practice and practice for hours and hours and never once feel cramped in the wrists. And after a long day at the office, you might find yourself in the subway, hanging from a strap, feeling squeezed and tired, your body twisted because there's people in your way, and if you'd never been to Carola Speads' studio, you'd just want to scream because everything's so terribly cramped and noisy. Because you have mastered Physical Re-Education, though, that's not going to happen. You breathe and relax. You pay attention to what you're feeling. The cars are rattling. The subway slows down, crawls, speeds up, rumbles, rattles. Someone smells awful. Someone bumps into you. Somebody sneezes. And you're standing on your shaky spot in the crowded metal box, and you mindfully take another few highly satisfying breaths. Then you wiggle your way to the door and get off and you're completely relaxed and ready, Carola says, for more.

When her relationship to Charlotte became more difficult, late in 1948, Carola turned to another project. She was convinced that mindful breathing would help women give birth. Offering courses for pregnant women: that was her new concept. Her daughter Dorothea, 25 years old, always dependable, newly married, and pregnant for the first time, lay down on a mat and put her legs up on a wooden box. The camera clicked. Next pose. Dorothea sat up, placed her chest on the box, and pretended to rest. Click. Excellent advertising material.

Much later, in the 1960s, the breathing exercises developed by the French gynecologist Fernand Lamaze are going to spread all over the United States. Lamaze found his therapeutic ideas in Stalinist Russia. Not such an attractive place, it seems. Nonetheless, more and more Americans, women and men both, will start to breathe rhythmically, in the French/Soviet way, in order to prepare for birth. They will attend Lamaze courses and practice the "choo-choo" breathing, like a train engine, and the hissing "sss-sss" breathing and the techniques called "huff and puff" and "slump and blow."[16] One of the bestselling books from these years will be titled *Thank You, Dr. Lamaze*. There will be no book titled *Thank You, Mrs. Speads*. She's ahead of her time.

Now Carola begins another experiment. She asks her clients to rest on their stomachs. She asks them to close their eyes. They're working on how to fall asleep. You lift one leg. The left one, let's say. You let gravity do its work and ever so slowly let your leg come back down. Then you wait. And you breathe. You shouldn't forget, Carola reminds them, that breathing isn't just inhaling and exhaling. There's a pause in-between. Consider that. Then lift your leg again, the same one, and then let it sink down again. Wait. Breathe out. Pause. Breathe in. Lift the left leg again. Not the right one. The left one. Never change that leg. Do it again. And again. At some point it's going to happen. Your whole body will relax, ready to sleep, because it's working only on that one leg and on nothing else.

There are some particularly successful clients who doze off, right then and there, in the studio. Sometimes a highly motivated student is going to want to wake them up. Carola stops that. They need this, she says. It's fine to fall asleep during her classes. It was the same way in Berlin, back then, before the war, on Frau Gindler's grey wall-to-wall carpet in Kurfürstenstraße. When people finally awoke, Frau Gindler would ask: "Was it nice?"

Emma Lazarus' poem on the Statue of Liberty's base invites the "huddled masses" to America, migrants "yearning to breathe free."[17] But that isn't so easy. There was this Tuesday in Donora, Pennsylvania, in October 1948, when a cloud settled over the valley. Donora's zinc mills blew their exhaust into the air, and, because of the cloud, the fumes didn't leave the valley. Only after five days did the fog lift, and it turned out that it had killed 20 people and made thousands very sick.[18]

In New York, by the open sea, this can't happen. And then it does. In November 1953, clouds paralyze the city's pollution for days on end. Some experts say it's smog. Some say it's "smaze" or "smoze." Others call it "smag" because that combines "smoke," "haze," and "fog." And the smog, smaze, smoze or smag refuses to let go of New York. The skyscrapers disappear, the bridges, and the park. You can't breathe in the stifling air. You can't not breathe it in either. Your eyes burn, your throat hurts. Your coughs rattle, your head aches. Asthma breaks out. New Yorkers call department stores and ask for gas masks. Unavailable. They call the fire department, asking them to do something. There's nothing that could be done. This city is prepared for nuclear attacks, but not for bad air. The *New York Times* suggests that its readers feel grateful they don't live in Donora, Pennsylvania. And yet dozens die in the smag.[19]

Carola and Charlotte had worked together for more than ten years. And then, when the 1950s had just begun, Charlotte told Carola that all she thought of were her clients' bodies. Their backs, their necks, their eyes, their breathing. What about the entire person, though? Why did Carola ignore the mind? Later, after they're no longer speaking to one another, Charlotte will tell others that Carola responded with a silent gesture. She rubbed her thumb and index finger together. Treating people's bodies: that was where the money was. According to Charlotte, her new enemy, that summed up Carola's mindset.

They became rivals on the mindfulness market. They still are, now, in 1954. But it's Charlotte and not Carola who has started teaching at the New School for Social Research, home of some of New York's most eminent refugee intellectuals. Philosopher Erich Fromm, Charlotte's client, has gotten her the job. How does this make Carola feel? It's not too hard to imagine. Like Charlotte, Carola had an affluent life in Berlin, and this year, almost a decade after the war, she can't buy Christmas presents because she still hasn't made it in New York. Charlotte has pulled through, even though she's so much less ladylike and her German accent so much rougher.

Carola writes a letter to Berlin, to Frau Gindler, about how unfair it all is. How she hadn't objected to Charlotte living in the studio they had rented as a teaching space only. How Charlotte had moved in with her and Otto when she was sick, how Otto and Carola had treated her like family and had always been there for her when she was so terribly depressed and how eventually Charlotte had shown Carola her "monstrous jealousy" and "bottomless hate."

Now the straws. Carola's clients hold them between their lips. They're breathing in through their noses and breathing out through the straws. She lets them do this for ten minutes and then for another ten minutes. For beginners, twenty minutes can seem like a very long time. You think about this and that. Your stomach rumbles. A leg goes numb. Time stands still. Your back hurts. All this is part of the experiment.

Carola sits and watches the breathers. The clients see: This is a woman who leads a completely mindful life. She probably doesn't squeeze her body into a subway car very often. And even if she did, she wouldn't mind. Some clients think that she spends her entire mindful life in this studio, ceaselessly enjoying the breezes coming in from the park.

But there's something her students may not realize. To succeed on the mindfulness market, she needs to appear as a model of inner peace. It's the only way she can attract clients. She can't show that her neck hurts or that she has financial worries. The Charlotte Problem: a secret. And she also won't or can't let them see the monstrous, indescribable darkness of her family history. Nor Dorothea's kidney problems and allergies and how her daughter almost suffocated, her life just barely saved. Ten days Dorothea spent in the hospital, and Carola had to take care of the boys in the busiest time of the year. Plus, Carola thinks of herself as fat. And she's tired, all the time. Menopause. She needs to give a lecture for massage experts, about relaxation, and another one for a group of psychoanalysts and another one, for a Jewish organization. They want her to talk about inner balance. She's looking at the breathers and their straws and she thinks about how she will need more students to make a living. In a letter to Frau Gindler she writes that she's "at the end of her rope." She can't take it anymore. She reads newspaper articles about the wave of antisemitism in the Soviet Union. She writes to Gindler "that we're only at the beginning of the horror and it's about to start now."

Then the Physical Re-Education expert decides that was enough breathing for the time being. She asks the clients how the experiment felt. Some respond. Some don't. She tells them in her relaxed, relaxing voice: Good. Keep working.

And she can't get over the fact that Frau Gindler doesn't take her side in the conflict with Charlotte. Gindler doesn't even comment. And to think that Charlotte had actually attended only two Gindler courses before 1933, two, only two, and that she never really got the point? And that, in 1952, Charlotte, because she's the more successful mindfulness teacher here in New York, and could afford the plane tickets, had gone to Germany and taken another Gindler course, her third, and she had then returned to perform as the one true Gindler disciple over here, in the United States? Carola reflects on all this in the long air mail letters she writes to Frau Gindler. She asks her for a confirmation letter that she was her assistant in Berlin and Frau Gindler says she doesn't write such letters. Carola explains that in the United States, "a country addicted to propaganda," having been someone's personal assistant needs to be documented. Frau Gindler still won't write that letter.

If the course ends as it usually ends, some students ask "Already?" and they look at a smiling Carola, who compliments them on their good work. It's a given, however, that the course really is over now, even for the most passionate clients. You don't involve Carola in an extended conversation. If someone cried in class, this does occur, Carola will talk to that person, briefly, calmly, and encourage them to seek professional help. You can't expect more from her. The students get up and put their mats into the corners of the room and they leave the room and on their way to the dressing rooms some peek into the kitchen, which seems a bit cold and empty. They take the elevators down and then they breathe in the air on Central Park West and there are cars and cabs and the rocks and the trees. They go back to the subway, or they walk back to work, or back home, and if they feel like most of Carola's students, if the straw experiment has worked for them, then they feel elated. As if they could breathe more freely. Take in more air. Meanwhile, ten floors up, Carola prepares for her next class.

2. Wandervögel

According to Carola Joseph, 16, future breathing expert, a woman named Grete Lubowski is the greatest math teacher anyone could imagine. Carola is a student at a girl's school in a Berlin neighborhood called Westend. It's the last year of World War One. 24 years later Frau Lubowski will go underground in Berlin to avoid deportation to the death camps. She'll be in hiding for two years. Now, in 1918, she's only six years older than most of her students, and she lets them call her "Grete." Because she's still a university student, Grete's stint is swiftly over, and Fräulein Dr. von Kühne will be teaching math from now on. That doesn't make anyone happy.

"Grete is a wonderful person," Carola notes in her diary on April 15, 1918. Like most German girls, she also keeps a poetry notebook that she circulates among her friends and people she admires. It is the custom to fill one of its empty pages with a particularly beautiful poem and then give the book back to the owner. She hasn't managed to hand her book to Grete, so Grete invites her over and they talk for three hours. Carola notes that Grete is a "straightforward, honest, intelligent human being with a sense of humor." Grete tells Carola about her year at the University of Heidelberg and about an "affair" she's had with one Fräulein von Probst. It is unclear what exactly that word means to them. Grete and Carola talk so much that there isn't even time for Grete to write something in the poetry journal. Grete operates on the principle, Carola writes, "to be outspoken about everything." And now Grete is even considering going on a hiking tour with Carola and her friends.

Carola is an avid diarist. Even when she was just nine years old she wrote about all the details of her life: how she had diphtheria and folded 112 paper birds on her sickbed, how she got a postcard from her father, away on a business trip, the owner of an animal feed factory, about her mother who brought her magazines, bread rolls and some caviar, and Aunt Bernhardine who sent a letter, and about how all the 112 paper birds she had folded were later burned for fear they could have carried the virus. She is an excellent observer. She can describe exactly what it feels like to rest on a meadow in the woods and to keep your eyes closed in the sun. To open your eyes and look at white cherry blossoms adrift on the dark water of a pond. And how much fun it is after a day out in the country to take the train back to Berlin with your fellow hikers and tell each other the silliest jokes.

And now she writes about what a complete joy it is to look forward to a long May weekend. Grete has confirmed. They will go to Gatow, a village on the river Havel. They will spend three days there. What a prospect: three days of hiking with Grete Lubowski.

In the early 20th century, young Germans generally hike a lot. Tens of thousands have joined the "Wandervögel" movement. "Birds of passage" comes to mind as the literal translation. "Avid hikers" would be more precise. Young Wandervögel are roaming through the forests. They're sitting at campfires. They're sleeping in barns. In these barns, or in meadows, in the woods, or maybe back home, they're writing lots of poetry about nature. They're feeling young and free but they're keeping their distance from the working class and revolutionary leftist ideals. They stress how "pure" and "patriotic" their movement is.[20]

The birds of passage are part of a larger social current which will later become known as the "life reform" movement. The reformers aim to discover nature – both around them and within them. Getting to the first kind of nature is easy. Take the train, get off, start walking. The path to nature within you seems more complicated. It leads to your own body, experienced in a mindful way. You need to feel what's going on inside. You need to breathe and think about how you take in air.

Writers associated with the life reform movement notice contemporaries whose bodies appear like "the saddest prison of the soul." They read modern cities as "piles of stones" that make the masses unhappy, lonely, ill, and nervous. Life reformers aim to create a newer, freer, happier type of human being. Some advocate expressive dance, some yoga, some "rune gymnastics" (which resembles yoga, except that it's meant only for "Germanics" and places great value on having "Aryan blood"). Life reformers promote nudism, body building, vegetarianism, or the philosophies of the Mazdaznan movement, formed, their spokesman claims, seven millennia earlier in Tibet and now led by Dr. Otoman Zar-Adusht Ha'nish, born as Otto Harnisch in West Prussia. He emphasizes that, as the son of a Persian princess, he is particularly well suited to save humanity, which he sees as "degenerated" by "racial mixing." The New Human Being, Otto/Otoman Hanisch/Ha'nish claims, should be pure. From a mail-order business much closer than Tibet, you can order Mazdaznan underwear and Mazdaznan rectal cleaning tools.[21]

In comparison to these variants of life reform, hiking seems conventional. But the girls out in the woods and fields are a problem, at least for male observers. One of the older, anti-feminist Wandervögel sees "the usual suffragette logic" in the mere thought that women could join the hiking movement.[22] Young women hike regardless. They don't wear gloves. That's provocative. They don't take purses either. They use backpacks. They don't take parasols, they don't take umbrellas, their dresses are loose. They want to see the world. Carola's one of them.

Then disaster unfolds. Yes, Carola and her friends do go on a hiking trip with Grete, from May 21 to May 23, 1918. Grete, however, while sleeping in the same room as Carola, never talks to her once. This wonderful human being only has eyes for somebody else: Carola's best friend Vesta. Even Vesta notices this. Once they're back from the trip, Vesta explains to Carola how nice that was, but how unfair, surely, for Carola. Vesta is a very spontaneous person. When she feels happy, she can almost faint. And she feels happy a lot. People often give Vesta flowers, extraordinarily often, really, Carola notes in her diary. "I am so happy anyway," Vesta tells Carola when they talk about Grete. "I don't even need all this." Then

Vesta and Carola kiss. But that doesn't change anything, and Carola later writes an accusatory letter to Grete Lubowski, a letter which sees multiple drafts. It's a letter she never should have sent. That is what Grete Lubowski tells her in a very concise response.

Vesta will eventually marry a zoologist. He will die at a young age – a hunting accident. He was after wild boar. Vesta marries again: an ornithologist this time, who, in 1960, receives one of the highest medals of communist East Germany.[23] Grete Lubowski graduates with a teacher's diploma and marries one Walter Draeger, a businessman, and she goes on to work as a teacher at a school in Berlin. Generations of students love her, until, in 1933, she is fired from her job because she's Jewish. In 1934 the new system creates an option for any "Aryan" Germans wishing to get divorced from their Jewish spouse. Walter Draeger takes this option. Newly single, Grete Lubowski works for a Christian-Jewish aid organization and takes up sculpture as a hobby. She then teaches in a Jewish school until she is forced to work in a Siemens & Halske factory. In 1942, she goes underground to avoid deportation, and late in July 1944, she is arrested, probably because some Berliner has denounced her. On August 10, 1944, she is forced onto a transport to Auschwitz. She will not survive.[24]

To her parents, in the early 1920s, Carola's plans for life after school seem scandalous. Paula Joseph, her mother, comes from a generation of women still wearing corsets. These women took the band that tightened the apparatus, tied it around a door handle, and then moved away from the door to make the corset as tight as possible. They kept moving even if the tightness already took their breath away. Carola's mother wants her daughter to lead a freer life, but not the kind of life that Carola has in mind. Carola's father Eduard started small as a fruit salesman, then moved on to grains. He thinks his daughter should study chemistry, start at his company, and at some point take over one third of it. If she doesn't get married first.

Everything about her scandalous plans began with the Wandervögel. Some of their group mentors kept talking about these "hours" they were taking. Apparently, these were lessons in something important, new, and fulfilling. They didn't tell them anything else and so the junior Wandervögel kept asking and wouldn't let up and finally discovered what these hours were all about. The mentors were doing gymnastics with an instructor named Anna Hermann. So the younger Wandervögel also made an appointment with Frau Hermann. They took off their dresses and put on bathing suits, held each other's hands, jumped about, kept their balance, stood on their tiptoes, and learned from their instructor that each body contained its "pure form." An ideal slumbered within it. Gymnastics, Frau Hermann says, is about finding that ideal.

Carola and her friends are certainly not the only Germans doing gymnastics in the early 20th century. There's the Ling System, which promises good posture, the Sandow System for athletes, the Mensendieck System for women. Mensendieck says you can get spare parts for every machine, but not "for the body machine."[25] This makes so much sense to people that "mensendiecken" becomes a verb in the German language. But most people doing gymnastics at home follow the Danish Müller Program. Müller's book *My System* has sold hundreds of thousands of copies. His readers try rubbing exercises. If they're particularly loyal, they buy tickets for Müller's lectures. On stages across Germany, Müller presents his rubbing, dressed in very small bathing trunks or in no trunks at all.[26]

Frau Hermann is different. She's more patient and personal than most gymnastics instructors. She doesn't have a "system." That, in fact, is the whole point. You move around. Or you rest. It always depends. On you. In Frau Hermann's studio Carola is lying on the floor between the other students. She breathes in, she breathes out, and she has the clear sense that she needs to help other people understand this. There's no question about it.

Her mother will not have her daughter consider a career in a bathing suit. And Carola gives in. She plans to study biology and talks to a professor. Along the way, though, something must have gone wrong. He treated her badly. Was it because she's a woman? Was it because she's Jewish? The details are unclear. She then settles for the humanities and enrolls at Berlin University to study German, English, and Philosophy. Her mother lectures her about the Wandervögel business. She'll never find a husband in that crowd, Paula Joseph says, and Carola's standards of what a man should offer are far too high anyway. Carola listens and takes notes. Then she decides to spend a year in Freiburg, in 1921/1922. Freiburg is a long way from Berlin and the Joseph family home. She studies at the university and goes to the movies and takes gymnastics lessons with a teacher trained in the "Loheland system," a method practiced in the nude.[27] She puts her clothes back on and goes on hiking trips in the Black Forest with fellow students and one of the hikers seems to have spent more time with her than the others. He's a law student named Felix Joachimson who will go on to become a famous writer in Berlin. His breakthrough: the comedy *How Will I Be Rich and Happy?* Later, under his new name, Felix Jackson will have quite the Hollywood career and live his life by the principle of never speaking a word of German again.[28]

Fig. 3: Hiking in the Black Forest. On the left: Carola Joseph.

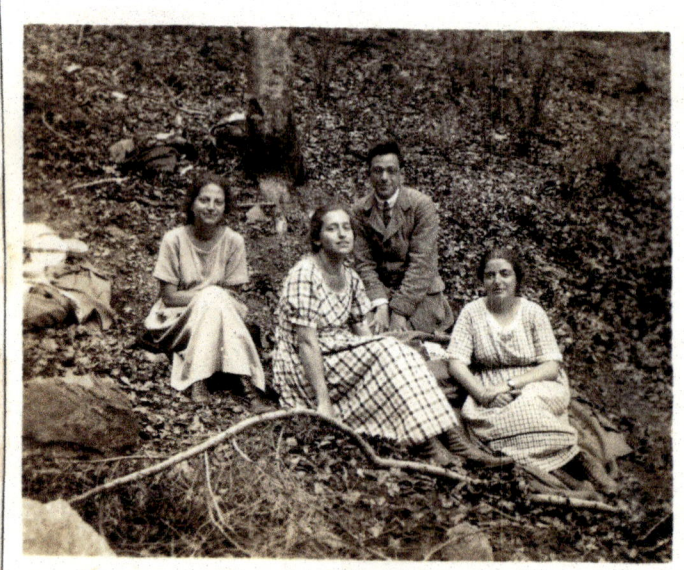

For some reason that she doesn't explain, Carola moves back to Berlin in 1922. She returns to Frau Hermann's studio floor. And she breathes. Everything begins with breathing. You must train your breathing and strengthen it before you turn to your body. First you learn the rhythm of breathing, then the force of breathing, then the balance of breathing and movement.

All the German gymnastics instructors of the time, and there are hundreds of them, have their own philosophies and principles and like to stress the enormous mistakes other gymnastics instructors make. What unites them all, nonetheless, is that they aim to bring body and mind into harmony. And they all emphasize rhythm. That's one of the buzzwords of these new times. The bodywork experts aren't talking about the rhythms of jazz or machines, but about the rhythms of nature: low tide and high tide, light and darkness, breathing in, breathing out.[29] Anna Hermann's colleague Clara Schlaffhorst is absolutely convinced that the "being and nonbeing of the entire German people" depends on the right and natural way of breathing. Across Germany, Schlaffhorst sees suffering and decay and "psychopathic children." But she knows what will help: breathing exercises according to the Schlaffhorst method. All the children trained by her, she says, had turned into "real giants."[30]

Anna Hermann, more of a realist, teaches the "vertical structure of the body," the "sense of direction," balanced musculature, and the "improvement of deformities." To Hermann, the pendulous abdomen and the humpback count as "deformities," as do bow-legs, knock-knees, and protruding shoulder blades. She's leading people toward "pure" movement. After 1933, in a new era, Anna Hermann will perform her gymnastics before Nazi leaders.[31] Now, a decade earlier, she offers Fräulein Carola Joseph an apprenticeship position. Carola enthusiastically accepts. Her mother still can't think of anything more embarrassing than a daughter prancing around half-dressed. And just imagine concerning oneself with other people's flat feet. But Carola won't be stopped.

When she isn't studying bowlegs, knock-knees, flat feet, and breathing, she goes to see the most famous expressionist dancers of her time. On

Berlin stages, the Falke sisters contort their bodies like snakes. There's Mary Wigman, so full of energy that she doesn't even need music. She moves around in complete silence. There's Harald Kreutzberg, his head shaved, his face masked. These dancers are inventing a new language of the body, ecstatic and abstract. Men are dancing so tenderly and softly that you could think they were women; women are dancing as powerfully as if they were men. You can't differentiate between dance and gymnastics anymore, either, but it doesn't matter, because now, in the 1920s, such categories seem irrelevant. It's all about harmony. In moving rhythmically, people say, the body becomes spiritual, and the spiritual turns physical.[32]

In 1925, Carola Joseph, a licensed gymnastics instructor, appears in a blockbuster film. To one critic it's "one of the most important creations since the beginning of cinematography." To another it's "un-German and disgusting." *Achieving Strength and Beauty* shows a spectacular panorama of sports, dance, and gymnastics. It features men and women, dressed and undressed, athletes and performers, and in one scene six representatives of the Hermann school, Carola is one of them, emerge from the woods dressed in white bathing suits. Hand in hand, they run wiggly lines around a clearing. They form a circle and together move this way and that, toward the camera and away from it and then back into the woods.

Inspired by the success of *Achieving Strength and Beauty*, a magazine sends a photographer to Anna Hermann's institute. Again, there's a lot of running around and a tug-of-war contest as well. Later that year, Frau Hermann asks Carola to give a lecture in her place, and before or after Carola delivers her talk, she performs the "Walk with Sounds." Carola may also have appeared at an event marking the "Day of the Horse." After a lecture about riding and a film about the "German crossbreed," Anna Hermann and her group, so the program says, showed rhythmic gymnastics and dances.

In 1926 Carola's students write to congratulate her on her 25th birthday. They call her "our dear class mama." One Dr. Blumenfeld wants to send his 18-year-old daughter to take classes with her. But he needs Frau

Joseph to promise that she'll "achieve something noteworthy in about six to eight weeks." One of her students hopes her instructor will be able to grade their papers without getting sick from reading them. Another one sends greetings from a German beach. She's doing gymnastics there, while breathing "sea air mixed with cow dung." A colleague writes to her because she wants to discuss "parallel feet positioning."

Fig. 4: Anna Hermann's students.

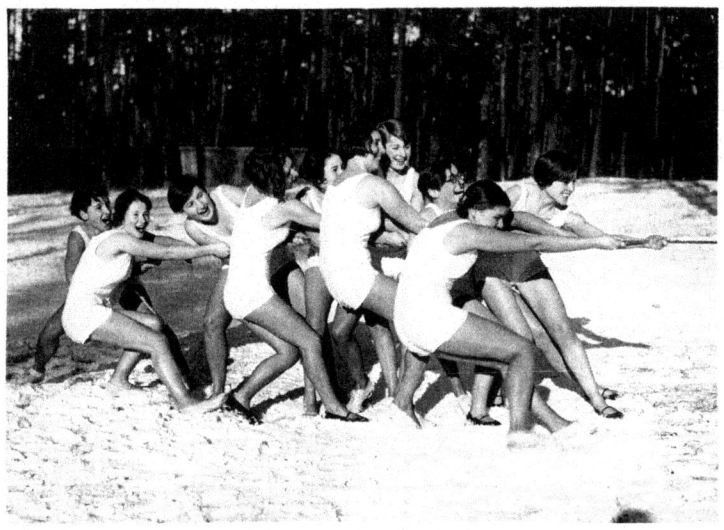

One letter could be more important than the others. At the offices of a Munich publishing house – Pössenhofer – an acquisitions editor with an illegible signature tells her that his press is looking for "seasoned authors" in the field of sports. He sends a stamped addressed envelope. Carola asks him to describe his request in more detail. The editor responds and asks her whether she would like to send Pössenhofer a manuscript. Half a century will pass before she finally gets a book done.

Carola is a teacher who wants to keep learning. And when it seems she can't learn all that much from Frau Hermann anymore, she hears about Elsa Gindler. A woman of legend. A new kind of gymnastics teacher. A teacher unlike anyone else.

In 1920s Germany a story circulates about Gindler: that she single-handedly cured herself of tuberculosis, a disease for which no cure exists. There are new ways to diagnose it, certainly, and there are new lung hospitals and sanatoriums for the rich. For the poor in the cities, though, little can be done. If you live in a dark, damp tenement, you're likely to catch it. You start coughing, that's the first phase, then your cough gets worse, the second stage, and you cough up yellowish green phlegm, then blood, or blood and phlegm, you lose weight, you're always tired, you have trouble breathing, and then you fade away.[33] Elsa Gindler, having grown up in poverty, had tuberculosis, and she knew what to do. Every day she left the damp flat she lived in and climbed the stairs to the attic and then she sat there, in the dry attic air, and breathed that air in. That's how she cleaned her lungs. She felt which lung the disease sat in, and she mindfully breathed into that part of the lung, strengthening it, and then moved on to the other part. And then her tuberculosis went away. Because she breathed.

Carola hears that Gindler will be teaching a course on the island of Sylt. She registers for the course. She takes days off from the Hermann school. She boards a train. Whether Gindler really beat tuberculosis is hard to say, but it's certainly true that she liberated herself from German class constraints. First she worked in a factory, and then as a maid, then she completed an apprenticeship as an accountant, worked as an accountant, didn't like that, worked as a stenographer, didn't like that either, joined a vegetarian club, organized women's groups and folk dance circles, explored music, painting, theater, Swedish gymnastics, fell in love with a man named Bernd, wanted more than friendship from him but didn't get it, read a book called *Harmonious Gymnastics*, and finally knew exactly what she wanted.[34] One year after Gindler's death, in 1962, her former students will meet in Israel to plant trees in her memory. Gindler helped save Jewish lives in Nazi Germany.[35]

2. Wandervögel

Carola may have heard about Gindler's famous lecture, held at the largest German gymnastics congress ever. Two thousand people were present in Düsseldorf, in 1926, and Gindler walked onto the stage and opened her talk by stating that her goal as a gymnastics teacher was not to teach gymnastics. She just wanted to make people concentrate. Unlike Frau Hermann, Gindler isn't looking for "pure form." Unlike Frau Schlaffhorst, she doesn't plan to save the nation. Gindler explores everyday situations. A married couple fighting. An office worker whose boss suddenly appears next to their desk. In such moments, Gindler says, breathing stops, or becomes far too intense, and the whole person turns self-conscious, anxious, unfocused. But even knowing that you're tightening up in such instances, Gindler says, can lead you out of the crisis. Mindfulness shows the way.

On the train to Sylt, Carola runs into Gindler. They talk. Gindler tells Carola how pretty her hair is. And on the island, Carola watches Gindler teach. She notices that Gindler notices everything. She makes them walk in the dunes and swing their bodies and she spots immediately when someone has a muscle that's causing them problems. The women go to the beach and do leap-frog jumps. Gindler registers what's working and what isn't, and suggests what people could do, and she always uses the right words. Gindler still claims that she can't really teach anyone anything and that she only wants to make you more intelligent.[36] Here on the island, she says, it's easy to loosen up. Of course. They're on vacation here. The true challenge is in the everyday. Gindler wants you to conduct experiments everywhere, always. How do you breathe while brushing your teeth? How do you breathe when you put on your socks? When you're eating? You need to ask yourself these questions. You need to do the research.

Carola takes the train back to Berlin. She's still Frau Hermann's assistant and this specific boss doesn't really believe in research. Carola can't stop thinking about Gindler. Everything is so different with her. Her work isn't about knock-knees and how to correct them. It's about being a person. It's about growing into someone who's "wholly there."[37] Frau Hermann and Carola tend to have unfriendly discussions now, about this detail and that.

In 1927 Carola's on her own and running a gymnastics studio in her parent's Berlin apartment. She keeps balls there, pillows, a broomstick, and a mug with straws in it.

One of Carola Joseph's clients is a girl named Ruth Hirschfeld. She complains of back pains. Later, in New York, she will become a famous psychoanalyst, under her new name Ruth Cohn, but at this point she is just a 15-year-old Berlin kid who sees her 25-year-old gymnastics instructor walk into the room, a "very slender, very pretty, very young woman" with a "beaming" smile. "Curly hair like an angel." That's how Ruth will remember Carola.

Ruth wants to do everything she can to please her teacher. But she realizes that isn't so easy. Carola asks her to sit on a pillow and to see what sitting feels like. Don't imagine what it feels like, Carola says. Feel it. Then she puts the broomstick on the ground before Ruth. She asks her to walk on it. It's not about being able to do it, she tells her. Again: It's about feeling what it's like. Ruth is an ambitious, competitive girl. She wants to balance on the broomstick all the way. She doesn't feel all that much. And when Carola wants her to breathe through a straw, she doesn't really get that either. The teacher tells her not to breathe in any special way. Just to let her breath escape. Ruth still doesn't get it. What she'll always recall, however, is that this teacher talked to her, the adolescent, as if she were an adult, even about sexuality. That, Carola told her, was something one should expect, but didn't need to rush.[38]

Carola takes courses with Elsa Gindler: Mondays and Wednesdays, 7-8 p.m., Kurfürstenstraße, Berlin. 15 women are sitting on the floor in a semi-circle. Their instructor invites them to look around and share what they notice. The women let their eyes wander here and there and then they report back. Not that there's all that much to say. Now Gindler tells them to sit with their eyes closed, to open them whenever it feels right, and to then look around once more and report back again. Everyone says that they noticed so much more. It's the transition from not-seeing to seeing that makes them mindful. They register the light and the colors of the room, and the high ceilings and they note that the windows really need to be cleaned.[39] They put blindfolds over their eyes and explore the room with their feet. Then they talk about how that felt. They crawl through rows of chairs and talk about that. They crawl over each other. Gindler watches and comments, but she doesn't criticize. They swing their chests. Their arms hang loose. They notice that the neck can let go.

It is unclear what cultural camp Carola Joseph, Elsa Gindler, and the other women belong to. In polarized 1920s Berlin, two world views collide. There are Germans who love modern furniture, cocktails, fast-paced music – and those that see all these things as indications of the decline of German culture. "Girl" is a popular word in German now. If you use it in English, instead of "Mädchen," it shows how modern you are. But these mindfulness students are definitely not the "Gindler girls." They don't sip cocktails. They don't build Bauhaus chairs. And they don't produce avant-garde art. They are housewives, actresses, medical doctors. One of them, Lily Ehrenfried, runs a practice for sexual counseling in Prenzlauer Berg. As a group, they don't fit into any of the categories for women of this period.[40]

Gindler says that not being stressed is a "condition of the highest reactive potential."[41] Her students are lying on their stomachs and relaxing their legs. Gindler notes: "Talked again about the connection to sexual organs. Bring sexual hygiene products for males." She notes on October 17, 1927: "Rubbers! Didn't get done." And on November 3: "Repeated Rubbers. Got it." The women let their legs hang loose and allow them to react to this kind of looseness. They feel how their pants are moving up their legs. They put their hands on the floor and let their pelvises sink down. They do somersaults over chairs. Gindler writes on October 19: "discussed at length that breathing is wonderful etc."[42]

Gindler and her students are withdrawing from the city, from modern Berlin. They only seem to care about their own breathing, their own bodies. They don't address mass unemployment, poverty, the housing crisis.[43] They come to Gindler's studio to find peace and quiet. In the late 1920s that in itself could seem like a reactionary concept. Even paying attention to your own body could appear like a right-wing idea, because the leaders of the nationalist movement keep praising the "organic," in contrast to "artificial" mass culture.

But it all depends on what you're looking for. In the quiet of Gindler's place, the women are only searching for themselves and not for not some life-saving force for all Germans.[44] They aren't interested in the "Volk." They're doing research on specific experiences, and they photograph and film their experiments: the Before, the After. In doing so, they produce a modern archive of the body. Gindler's collection of photographs and films, a marvelous multimedia project, will be destroyed in the war that is to come.[45]

Carola's father dies in 1928. The family mourns and all the business issues need to be arranged. Carola can't count on her brother Heinz. He has broken all ties to the family. Her mother seems "completely helpless." Carola arranges everything. She has no clue how these things work, but she deals with them and applies what she learned from Gindler – and from herself. Just to "feel what needs to happen." That is her goal. She gets things done.

There aren't many documents on what's going on in Carola Joseph's life at this point. She's pushing thirty. She writes about a lot of "unsettling events." Her brother marries a woman named Alice Philipps on January 17, 1929, and they get divorced a few months later. In April 1930 Carola takes a trip to Italy. She wants to stay for at least half a year "to find [herself] again." She returns to Berlin after just three months because she needs to deal with her father's business matters. She moves into a friend's apartment, then into her mother's place. And then her mother and Carola stop talking, because Carola has started looking for a place of her own. Or is it the other way round: Is she looking for a place because she just can't live with her mother?

From December 1, 1930, onward, Carola Joseph, 29, runs her own "private school for gymnastics" from her new apartment in Offenbacher Straße. She's one of 1,150 members of the German Gymnastics Association. The fact that she's an official member means that she's an expert and not a quack. Not everyone can join the Association, only those educated in gymnastics, pedagogy, and in "matters of the body and the soul." The Association firmly believes that the professional way of doing gymnastics should be fundamentally different from "superficial imitations," from "fashionable" bodywork "of a sugary, overly disciplined or art-addicted kind." The Association emphasizes that training rooms must be "hygienically perfect" and "satisfyingly lighted." Adults may practice in an undressed state if they find themselves in gender-segregated groups, but only if there are "factual reasons" to take off their clothes. Practicing in the nude is fine, the Association says, if the students are children.

The psychoanalyst Otto Fenichel now takes Gindler courses. As a schoolboy in Vienna, any kind of sport made him suffer. Not much has changed since then. After the lessons, his muscles ache, his tendons, his joints. But the headache that has plagued him since forever has suddenly disappeared.[46] He's a convert. In a lecture at the Berlin Psychoanalytic Society, he elevates Gindler's teachings to the same level as psychoanalysis. Both these methods, Fenichel explains, disrupt automatic processes, be they psychological or physical. Both methods lead people to a more conscious life and make the self seem less "small and weak." He's enthusiastic about Gindler's search for "efficient movements." These are movements, he says, of people reflecting their own lives. Maybe because Fenichel praises her so generously, his colleagues Erich Fromm and Wilhelm Reich also join Gindler's classes.[47]

In 1931 Carola Joseph starts seeing a psychoanalyst. She reads a lot of Freud at this time. She's good friends with Claire Fenichel, Otto's wife, who's also a gymnastics teacher. It's characteristic of these times that most psychoanalysts are male and undisputed authority figures, whereas gymnastics, the less renowned field, is much more open to women.

In *Zeitschrift für Psychoanalyse*, Claire's husband posits that the act of breathing is an act of empathy. Every person who identifies with another person doesn't just imitate this person, but also breathes like them. You change your inhaling and your exhaling because you want to be close to the other. And if there's a moment of surprise, something new, then people stop breathing, because the self uses breath to figure out whether it should feel afraid or not.⁴⁸ In a later essay on the "psychopathology of coughing," Otto Fenichel will analyze the nervous breathing obstructions of public speakers. They cough, he says, because through speaking publicly they are satisfying their exhibitionism. That makes them feel guilty. So they cough. And the coughing attacks in the audience are unconscious yet aggressive disruptions of the performer at the lectern.⁴⁹

In early 1930s Berlin, Elsa Gindler plays a record. She tells everyone to roll around, on the floor, to the music. And everyone starts rolling, except for one woman. Carola's watching that student. She sees that this woman's body should certainly be able to roll. Nothing physical seems to be stopping her. Something else is in the way. Carola believes that psychoanalysis, not gymnastics, could help that woman find out what stops her from rolling.

Carola tells Gindler that she's seeing an analyst. Gindler doesn't have much time for the theoretical discussions the Freudians are involved in. She says these would "knot up the psyche."⁵⁰ She asks Carola whether she thinks that what she calls "our work" isn't good enough anymore. Carola says it's something else. She talks about the woman who didn't roll, who seemed to have a deeper problem. "She couldn't get across," Carola says. Gindler thinks for a minute and then says: "Yes, that's interesting." She seems to accept psychoanalysis. To Carola, that's an important moment.

And then she meets a man at a party. He's tall and dark-eyed and he has the same small mustache as the radically antisemitic future German leader. The man is fourteen years her senior. He's friendly. He's attentive. He's a Jewish Czech. German is his native language. He also makes his living with breathing and stress-relief: He runs a cigarette factory. Menthol cigarettes and so-called "Russian cigarettes." Kraj Orient, Kraj Club, Kraj Prima, Kraj Luxus and Kraj Cabinet. Advertisements say that these are "mixtures of a very special kind."

The dark-eyed man is a single father. His daughter is nine years old. Her mother died a few weeks after giving birth. Carola realizes what that means. She spent years getting away from her family. If she married this man, she'd be more than just his wife. She'd be a mother, too. She'd have to give up so much. And yet he does cut an elegant figure.

3. Notice What Is

In 1955 Otto and Carola Spitz have no idea that the Great Salad Oil Swindle will eventually shake up their world. They are a bit better off now than the year before. The elevator takes more and more students to the tenth floor. Carola teaches more one-on-one classes – these are much more lucrative for her. And Otto has left Fredo's failure behind him and the traveling salesman experience, too. He now works on Wall Street and manages the portfolios of other European refugees. He makes solid, conservative decisions. In March Carola writes to Elsa Gindler that she's planning to travel to Europe. "We won money on the stock exchange," she explains.

She returns to Germany for the first time after 1938. She spends some time in Berlin. Then she takes a Gindler course in a Bavarian village. Gindler and she both booked rooms in Gasthaus Zillibiller in Hindelang. They are living under the same roof, after all these years. Once the course is over, Carola takes a steam cure at Bad Reichenhall. She breathes in and she breathes out. There's salt in the water and in the steam, salt that's been trapped within the mountains for millions of years. Twenty years before, this town barred Jews from the spa facilities.[51]

Their neighborhood is changing. You don't notice it so much on Central Park West, but in the cross streets, things are different. Affluent families and their servants used to live in the brownstones. Then many wealthy New Yorkers moved to the suburbs and the town houses turned into tenements. Their new owners split them up into small apartments and rented them out, mostly to Puerto Ricans. Looking for jobs, looking for security, these are arriving in New York by the hundreds of thousands. Their landlords rip them off. Sometimes ten people live in one room.[52]

Some New Yorkers now perceive the Upper West Side as dangerous. When Otto and Carola have visitors, they tell them to walk along 86th Street to get to their building. There are bus lines along that street and it's always busy. 85th Street they advise against. When they're driving in their car, Otto and Carola Spitz always make sure the windows are up. Those among Carola's students who come from less tony neighborhoods feel that certain Upper West Side sophisticates might be overly afraid.

A violinist finds his way to the studio. He's having problems with his hands. When he's playing, he needs to hold them up, sometimes for hours, and then they turn lifeless and grey. Carola shows him a trick. It's a secret. And then he feels the blood rush back into his hands and knows how to do that trick again, whenever he needs it.

An oboist emerges from the elevator. She can't play the vibrato anymore. Carola watches her play and notices her strange posture. She has her swing her body forward. No vibrato. Backward. No vibrato. Then the oboist finds her balance point. There it is. The vibrato. They can hear it. The oboist just needs to stand the way her body and her breathing want her to. Then the vibrato will stay with her.

Carola loves students like this. But there are the other clients. There are these mothers, for instance, who feel exhausted because they can't find the right kind of dresses for their daughters and therefore urgently need to consult Mrs. Speads. Most people, it seems, just want to get rid of their pain, as quickly as possible. They don't want to explore. They just want help.

Right after the war, in 1947, she had the most motivated clients she's ever had, in Oak Ridge, Tennessee. In the Oak Ridge labs, scientists had produced the material for the bombs on Hiroshima and Nagasaki. Once the products of their work had been used, two cities destroyed, one war over and a new one, the Cold War, just begun, their patriotic research needed to produce more results.[53] Working with these scientists under pressure, Carola explored how to get rid of nervous tension. She showed them how a cramped-up person could bend forward, arms hanging to the ground, and how their fellow scientists, with light pats on the back, could manage to loosen up that specific body and the way it breathed.

No one was ever as focused on the work, she recalls, as these experts on nuclear weapons. And 251 Central Park West is her Oak Ridge. A research lab. Though few of her clients see that. They probably think she's some sort of physical therapist. Her mother may have been right: she's taking care of other people's flat feet. That's not what she wants.

Fig. 5: Breathing in the studio (Photographer: Carola Speads).

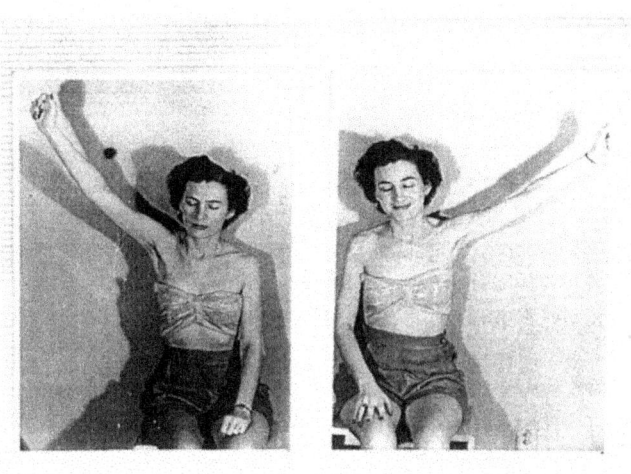

There are so many New Yorkers now who have trouble breathing. They have asthma and often it's intense. Gasping, wheezing, coughing, they show up in hospital emergency rooms. And they don't just arrive on days when the city's oppressed by smog (the term "smaze" hasn't really taken hold). Their crises are independent of the weather. African Americans and Puerto Ricans suffer the most. Harlem is the asthma capital.

What are the reasons? The debates are complex and often shaped by prejudice. Some scientists see asthma as a psychosomatic disease. They think that the illness is rooted in experiences of discrimination or inner-city violence. Others claim that the children of problematic parents are at greater risk of asthma. Over-protective mothers cause asthma in their children, some experts say, and others state that under-protective mothers do, too. And then there's "blatella germanica," the pest most prevalent in the New York slums. The cockroach triggers allergies which lead to asthma, and this observation prompts rumors that it's simply poor hygiene that causes the illness. In New York "cockroach" is a racist insult for Puerto Ricans. It's mostly white landlords, though, who let their tenements rot and thus create perfect living conditions for the cockroach.[54]

A German spa location named Freudenstadt – "Pleasure Town" – hosts a breathing congress in 1959. The names Gindler, Speads, or Selver don't appear in the program. A Dutch baron gives a lecture, Robert van Heeckeren, his sister a lady-in-waiting to Queen Juliana. The baron is a yoga teacher, and he shows slides illustrating "Breathing Questions for Woodworkers." He talks about men chopping down trees in Northern Norway. The baron has found out that these men sometimes take breaks and that they use these breaks to inhale deeply. 500 breathing experts listen. A doctor from Munich also speaks: Johannes Ludwig Schmitt. In some circles he's known as "Breathing Schmitt." He says that any sensation-mongering breathing instructor is no breathing instructor at all. A speaker named Otto-Albrecht Isbert complains about "the degenerate form of breathing" that every average "stressed-out, short-of-breath contemporary human being" will exhibit. During the Nazi years, Isbert was a very successful geographer. Now he has found a new calling. To his audience in Freudenstadt he recommends yoga to fight their degeneration, and perhaps some "light sniffling," through the nose.[55]

Carola writes to Elsa Gindler that her potbelly, after two months of dieting, has turned into a "cute little potbelly." She reports about her menopause and what it does to her glands. She talks about how happy she is when she menstruates again. It doesn't happen very often. Her neck keeps hurting, but that's something she can't change. Her everyday existence still doesn't seem as relaxing as one would expect from a relaxation expert.

Gindler sends her a document stating that, before 1933, Carola was "well-known as a successful gymnastics teacher in Berlin" and Carola sends the document, along with diplomas, letters, student and income records, prewar, wartime, and postwar, to the authorities in Berlin. On December 1, 1960 a decision is made there that the Federal Republic of Germany will pay monthly benefits and reparation money to Carola Spitz, "Jewish in the sense of the Nuremberg Laws."

In 1961 Adolf Eichmann sits in a bullet-proof cabin in a Jerusalem courtroom. On West End Avenue, Manhattan, Fritz Spitz, Otto's brother, Carola's brother-in-law, sits on the living room couch in the family apartment. He's watching Eichmann on the screen of the family's TV set.

Fritz and his wife first escaped from Vienna to Amsterdam, then to Marseille, then to Northern Africa. In Morocco they lived in a camp. Then they managed to get a passage across the Atlantic and arrived in the United States when it was almost too late. Fritz's daughter Frances says that life hardened her father. He will live in the United States for decades and when the telephone rings he'll always lift the receiver and bark: Spitz am Apparat! In German, of course. Why use any other language? His daughter Frances is so embarrassed. Other fathers, more American ones, lift the receiver and say: Hello. That sounds soft and smooth. Her family will always be different.

When his brother Otto dies, Fritz Spitz will respond to the news with nothing but a fierce intake of breath. He won't have words. When his wife dies, Fritz will acquire a new partner just a few weeks later. Not a partner he loves, he points out to Frances. The only woman he ever loved was his mother. He just needs a partner, he says, and that's that.

The former SS-Obersturmbannführer Eichmann, head of the "Referat für Judenangelegenheiten im Reichssicherheitshauptamt," answers another question about his role in the mass murder of the European Jews. And then Frances hears a loud bang and the sound of broken glass, because Fritz Spitz has picked up the living room lamp and thrown it at the TV, right at Adolf Eichmann. Spitz am Apparat.

On February 3, 1961, six advertisements for New York City television stores appear on page 11 of the German Jewish newspaper *Aufbau*. The article above these ads presents Carola's obituary of Elsa Gindler.

She states that Gindler's ideas have spread across the world and changed "modern education." She calls Gindler a "genius," but she also stresses her loyalty, her integrity, her honesty. She writes that Gindler sent food packages to former Jewish clients who'd been taken to concentration camps and that, up to 1938, Gindler taught Jews and Non-Jews together. After the war, Carola saw her as sick, impoverished, and tired, and then in a new, intense phase of creativity, "every working year more lucid than the one before." Carola stresses how happy Gindler was about the development of Israel as a "land of youth and the future." She paints the portrait of a powerful woman. "These were fascinating years," Carola writes, "and I remember her with woefulness and gratitude."

Carola and Charlotte don't talk anymore. Erich Fromm always books one private lesson per week with Charlotte, as does Fritz Perls, the founder of gestalt therapy. Charlotte has teamed up with Alan Watts, the most famous Buddhist in North America. They co-teach courses in New York and on Alan's houseboat in Sausalito, California. Charlotte's courses used to be called "Breathing" or "Eyes and Neck." Simple and straightforward. Now she teaches "Moving Quietness," or "The Unity of Opposites," or "The Tao at Rest and in Motion." She mixes German gymnastics and Buddhist mindfulness and American poetry. This new approach will make her a millionaire.

Carola's husband is the Wall Street trader Otto Spitz. Charlotte's new boyfriend is the bohemian Charles Brooks. He's the son of a Pulitzer Prize winner, a Harvard graduate, and a carpenter. Loves to dance, lives in a loft in the Village, throws the wildest parties there. Had a friend tell him about this woman whose teachings made the fist disappear that this friend had always felt in his stomach. Charles came along and listened to Charlotte. Do you feel where you're standing? she asked. He became her student, her lover, her partner. He replaces Alan Watts.

Charlotte has also renamed "the work." Gindler had always reminded them that the "work" was just "the work" and that there should never be another name for it. Charlotte begs to differ. She and Charles now teach "Sensory Awareness." In the winter they teach it in a Mexican village, in the spring on the Californian coast, in the summer on a Maine island. Because Charlotte's hearing's getting worse, it is Charles' task to listen to any questions students might have about "Sensory Awareness" and to relay these questions to Charlotte. But Charlotte does most of the talking anyway. She talks about grass and how every leaf of grass moves differently in the wind and how, in a similar vein, every sort of breathing is also different. And that you might want to think about being breathed and not so much about breathing. She tells her students that when you're doing the dishes, the dirty dishes are asking you to please wash them. If you're sensorially aware, you'll be feeling the warmth of the water and the texture of the dishes, their weight, and you'll also feel the room you're in and the air you're inhaling, and she says that your heart will then begin to smile. Just because you're doing the dishes.[56]

In the early 1960s, Carola and Otto have other problems. There's one Tino De Angelis, client of Ira Haupt, Otto's Wall Street firm. Tino De Angelis has found out that you can make a lot of money if you pretend to the world that you own a great deal of raw materials. Say: salad oil. If you possess – or say that you do – a lot of salad oil in gigantic tanks, then you can use that to borrow a lot of money. Of course, you'll have to prove that you really own so much salad oil. But that isn't a problem if you're Tino De Angelis and you keep tanks with water in them instead of oil. When someone shows up to check on things, you just put a little oil on the water, and because oil happens to stay on top, no one's going to notice, and you'll keep making money. Eventually Tino De Angelis will own more salad oil than the entire United States put together, in theory, and nobody notices, until somebody does, and the stock market almost collapses and the firm Ira Haupt, employer of Otto Spitz, 251 Central Park West, is barred from trading on Wall Street.⁵⁷ Otto, 76 years old, is going to have to look for yet another new career.

Susan Elrauch sings while she's doing the dishes. She's a teenager in Flatbush, Brooklyn. She dreams of being an opera singer. She does the dishes a lot. The neighbors hear her singing and tell her parents how talented she seems to be.

Susan's mother is a secretary. Her father works nights, sorting letters in the post office. During the day he's asleep. If he happens to be awake, he tells Susan she should stick with who she is. Flatbush doesn't have opera singers.

Because the neighbors insist, Susan eventually does take singing lessons. She begins a performing career. At the charity afternoons of Jewish welfare organizations, there's coffee and cake and then Susan takes her guitar and sings "Donna, Donna, Donna" or the "Moorsoldaten." Or "Tumbalalaika," about the young man who asks what can burn eternally and the girl who answers that it's love. "Libe kon brennen un nit ojfheren!" Susan gets a degree from City College, a BA in Political Science and History. But all she wants to do is sing. In the Village clubs, she sings folk songs, like that singer from Minnesota: Bob Dylan. Susan Elrauch has different plans for her voice than Dylan. And her singing teacher, a German refugee, pinpoints some technical questions. What's she going to do with the long passages, the ones for which she's really going to need her breath? And what about the not so perfect way she inhales? That's something she needs to work on. Her teacher recommends Carola.

Susan gets off the subway at 86th Street, Manhattan, takes the elevator, and when she walks into the dressing room, she can tell she's not in Flatbush anymore. Carola's clients are artists, academics, wealthy people. A very special crowd. But then Susan sits on that mat on the floor and the light is coming in through the window and she breathes, and watches Carola teach. She's captivated. It seems as if Carola was truly interested in her students' experiences. She doesn't just pretend. She really seems to want these people to feel changes occur within them. She looks at them in their bathing suits and swimming trunks and she wants them to get better. She's so completely different from the singing and piano teachers Susan knows. There's nothing authoritarian about her. She never says: Do it like this and not like that.

After the trial lesson, Susan feels high. There's so much oxygen in her blood. But she can't afford these courses. They're for the affluent classes, not for her. And then she does come back after all.

The Therapeutic Era begins with the building of a fence: in Big Sur, California, in 1961. Behind this fence, the Esalen Institute will grow. The fence deters the gay men who in pretherapeutic times met here for swims. Esalen offers seminars that promise a completely new way of thinking about what it means to be a human being. A yogi and a shaman are among the institute's staff. The founders are confident that they're helping to shape the biggest changes in humankind since the Renaissance. They develop concepts that move beyond psychoanalysis and behaviorism, ideas that can make people healthy, that allow them to grow and utilize their psychic potential. And if psychoactive drugs should help, then why not?

In the second year of Esalen's existence, the institute hires Charlotte Selver. She teaches mindfulness workshops with a view of the ocean. When she's still a beginner at Esalen, she takes LSD. It's her first time. She's in her mid-sixties. She announces that she will jump from the cliffs and fly over the Pacific. She doesn't. She's going to teach at this institute until she's 99 years old.

According to Esalen, there's a "divine spark" inside every human being. All you need to do is find it. An expert named Bernard Gunther appropriates Charlotte's method and transforms it into what will become known as the Esalen Massage. No kneading. Only tapping. Candles flicker. Oil drips. Gunther invents the "Gunther Sandwich," which involves naked people lying as close to each other as possible. There's also mutual shampooing.[58] Future historians will find that a "religion of no religion" developed in Esalen. A new era begins in which people pay for making spiritual experiences. Your bank account needs specific qualities if you want your divine spark to ignite.[59]

Fig. 6: A relaxation experiment in the studio (Photographer: Carola Speads).

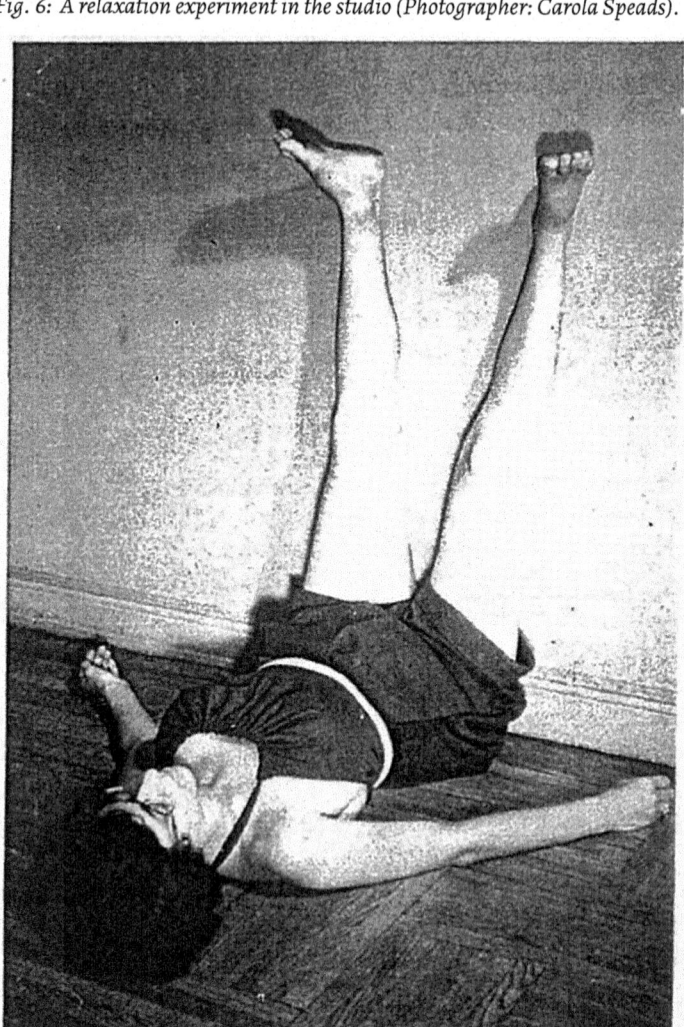

Nobody invites Carola to Esalen. She probably hears about Charlotte's ascent, her close relationships to the biggest names of her time, about Charlotte and Charles, the unconventional, dynamic, creative couple who fly back and forth between the coasts and Mexico. Otto and Carola also get on planes sometimes. They travel to the German Black Forest or Switzerland. They take walks there, hand in hand.

They no longer have financial worries. After the Salad Oil Crisis, Otto joined another company on Wall Street. He's going to be in business for a few more years. Carola cuts back a little on her teaching. Is she sacrificing her career for Otto? Would she like to do more? She rarely gives lectures anymore. She doesn't advertise her courses. When she takes the bus to Yorkville, she buys crossword puzzle magazines in German. It seems like she's letting go of "the work."

Susan from Flatbush does summer theater in Saratoga Springs. They do *Anything Goes* and *Marat/Sade*. She has supporting roles in these plays. Her father was very worried about his daughter's first summer of freedom, so he used his connections to make this period as unfree as possible. He called the post office in Saratoga Springs, talked to his colleagues there, and found Susan a room in an old lady's house in the suburbs. Now Susan is isolated from the immoral theater crowd.

She makes use of this solitary life. Every morning, she sits in her room and breathes as Carola Speads has taught her to. She pays attention to the air that streams into her body. She breathes in normally, not even all that deeply. She shuts her mouth, and she exhales through a very tiny gap. Ssssss. Or: Fffffff. This trains her diaphragm. She's sitting on her sit bones, another Carola teaching. That improves her posture. And then Susan gets a main part. In *Kismet*, she plays the beautiful young woman who falls immortally in love with the caliph, even though the caliph is set to marry at least one of the princesses of Ababu.

At family reunions, Frances, Carola's niece, watches her aunt and uncle and thinks they're completely old-fashioned. Otto always wears a suit, tie, and hat. The grey hat with the grey suit. The brown hat with the brown suit. Carola always wears dresses, never pants. A clear sign, to Frances, of her backwardness. (Carola's clients will later recall that Carola always wore pants, never dresses. A clear sign of how progressive she was.)

Now, in the late 1960s, if you're crossing Central Park West and you walk ahead into the green, you can smell marijuana clouds drifting over the grass. There are "Be-ins" and "Gay-ins." Naked couples disappear into the bushes and emerge a while later with changed facial expressions. In 1967 Martin Luther King Jr. leads 100,000 people through the park to protest the Vietnam War. Smoke rises from burned draft documents and smoldering US flags. Shouting in rhythmic unison, the protesters ask the American president how many people he killed today. From the elegant apartment buildings on Central Park West, letters are sent to the municipal administration, inquiring why certain rules of behavior don't seem to apply anymore.[60]

Frances listens to Carola and Otto talk, and she feels as though they're not interested in any of the issues of their time. In 1966 a task force publishes its report on air pollution in New York. Toxic gases are polluting the city: sulfur oxide, carbon monoxide, nitrogen oxides. The committee stresses that New York's survival is a pure stroke of luck. Were the city located in a valley, New Yorkers wouldn't exist anymore.[61] When someone asks Carola whether her breathing exercises might not be dangerous, given all that air pollution, she answers that the advantages of taking in oxygen are more beneficial than the disadvantages of pollutants.

There's no "political talk" with Otto and Carola, Frances says, no "community talk." The harbors close. The textile industry leaves the city, the printing industry. New York loses hundreds of thousands of jobs and almost goes bankrupt, fires teachers, garbage workers, social workers, cuts back spending for the subway, the busses, the police. There are about 1,000 murders per year. New York is caught in a state of ever more intense economic injustice. Some neighborhoods almost nobody can afford. That's where the elite hide out. Other parts of the city are mired in poverty and fear.[62] The air might be improving on account of the factories' departure and new anti-pollution laws. But the streets stink of garbage. People don't talk about these things at Spitz family reunions.

Then again, Frances' aunt does seem to be rather important. From time to time, she gives interviews. These don't address pollution, war, or the urban crisis; instead, Carola talks about how critical it is to change, every couple of days, from high-heeled shoes to flat-soled shoes and back again. This diversification will strengthen the thigh muscles. Carola also has recommendations for people sitting in orthopedically problematic movie theater seats. Place a handbag between your back and the seat back and it will do wonders for your posture. As your handbag is located behind you like that, place its strap between your behind and the seat. It will make your bag so much harder to steal.

Singer Susan returns to Carola's lessons. She will be her student for 32 years. In order to afford this luxury, she takes on additional jobs. She teaches English to recent immigrants, practices vocabulary, grammar, and irregular verbs with them, walks to the subway, rumbles to 86th Street, turns from teacher into student. "No expectations," Carola says. "Simply notice what is." The goal is to be interested. To be curious. "It's an experiment," Carola says. "Be open-minded." And she has such an agreeable voice.

Because her own voice isn't so bad either, the City Opera hires Susan. She is from Flatbush and has become an opera singer. Who would have thought? Certainly not her father.

In the opera dressing room, however, she suffers. It's a combination of stage fright and the fear of the first high C. It's altogether possible that she won't make the first high C tonight. Yes, it is possible. But then: Susan has Carola's experiments. She simply needs to find her breath. She gets up, all cramped up, and walks around, her arms raised. That way she's working with gravity, not against it, and blood flows from her arms and back down to her heart. She breathes in. She breathes out. And then she starts hopping, which Carola also recommends. In the belly of the opera Susan's hopping around, her arms still up in the air, hopping and hopping until the shoulder joints loosen up and she's made gravity's work so much easier. Decades later, she will concede that all this may only have served to take her mind off the first high C. But even if that was the case, Susan still says that Carola changed her life.

In the Studio of Physical Re-Education, there's now a basket containing authentic Japanese back tappers. Sometimes Bernice Selden gets tapped, an author of children's books and a member of the American Communist Party. Sometimes it's therapist Edith Kramer, sometimes art historian Philip Gould. He lifts his knee, against gravity. He lowers his knee, with gravity. He notices the light coming in through the windows. He moves his shoulder a little bit in one direction and then back again. And then he asks himself how that felt.

Carola says they shouldn't do anything heroic. Let the body do its own thing. Philip says that for an ambitious New Yorker like him, that's not so easy. But after class, he feels light as a feather. He leaves the studio, walks away from the building, a spring in his step, and after 90 Carola minutes views the world as a wonderfully friendly place.

In Berlin, in dialogue with Otto Fenichel, Carola Joseph wanted to understand what keeps people from living free, expressive lives. Then came the years of persecution. Here in New York, she has withdrawn into the studio, away from discussions, from language itself. She is silent a lot and her clients seem to like that. It gives her that ethereal aura.

In contrast to Carola, Charlotte Selver talks all the time. In her courses, too, clients lie around, trying to feel their own bodies with as much sensitivity as possible. While they're doing that, though, Charlotte presents one piece of wisdom after the other. She's teaching a course on breathing, for instance, and she says: Air is a guest that comes and goes. Or: My little cat is a wonderful teacher for me. Nobody seems to mind. In fact, people will start buying cassette tapes with audio recordings of Charlotte's courses.

Though Carola's so much more withdrawn, one day a journalist emerges from the elevator to get tapped with those Japanese tappers. She wants to be silent with Carola and write about the experience. What the journalist doesn't know: Her jaw is tense. Carola notices right away. The expert in charge of the Studio of Physical Re-Education begins an experiment designed to loosen it up, and that's exactly what happens: Minutes later the journalist's jaw feels so much looser. And Carola also notices that before the journalist does. The journalist is tremendously impressed with these observational skills, and reports from Central

Park West for the readers of *Mademoiselle* magazine, in May 1970. She quotes Carola's observation that Sensory Awareness, Charlotte Selver's method, really makes no sense at all. And she calls Carola a "guru."

Carola's grandson, Steven, receives a birthday package from his Omi. He starts opening the package. After three years in a Kibbutz, he has returned from Israel. His relationship to his grandmother is a bit fraught. As a teenager he protested when, year after year, his Jewish family gathered around a Christmas tree in 251 Central Park West. It felt like an insult to him. And he certainly isn't aware that she's a guru. When Steven thinks about breathing, he doesn't think of cocktail straws. He might think about the end of the Shabbat and how, to mark that moment, you breathe in the aroma of herbs – and about how Adam's creator breathed life into the first human being.

In Carola's package for Steven there's a Haggadah from the year 1781. It was printed in Amsterdam, an heirloom from her mother's family. You use the Haggadah at the Seder table, at dinner, the night before Pesach: as a collection of stories and a guide to the rituals. It's a book for children and for scholars. You can get caught up in the tales or theorize its contents. Because the Haggadah has to be placed on the table and because kids look at it, and because sometimes a glass of wine will get knocked over, these books often have stains and other blemishes.[63] The Haggadah that Carola gives her grandson is in remarkably good condition. It can't have been used much in the Spitz household. Probably not at all.

From now on Steven's grandmother will send him a book in Hebrew, from her library, on each one of his birthdays. He has no idea where she finds them. He's visited her apartment since he was a child and he's always been interested in Judaism, but he's never seen these kinds of books on her shelves. Freud's works in German and medical books, too, and monographs on cultural theory. Once, in her studio, he also held Anaïs Nin's autobiography in his hands, signed by the author, and he concluded that Nin might have found the time to breathe in Carola's studio, through a cocktail straw, who knows. But nothing in Hebrew. Only after Carola's death, when they clear out her Central Park West apartment, will they find these volumes, her grandfather's books, in a second row on Omi's shelves, hidden away from view.

In the 1970s therapeutic culture is spreading across the entire United States. The time of political movements seems to be over. Now it seems a bit old-fashioned to want to change the world. People try meditation and jogging, bioenergetics, acupuncture, tai-chi, or yoga. There's Rolfing, developed by Ida Rolf, there's Feldenkrais by Moshé Feldenkrais, and the Ilana Rubenfeld method. There's always somebody with a brand-new method. If you can afford it, there's Esalen.

Some people find this irritating. Historian Christopher Lasch sees a society without any sense of collective action. There are no societal visions in the therapeutic, Lasch posits, no political opportunities.[64] There's only mental health for the narcissistic self. The higher the standing of mindfulness, Lasch says, the closer the collapse of society.[65]

Then again, you could also use the trend for your own purposes. There's Peter Workman, for instance, a man of Lasch's generation. In 1968 he starts his own publishing house. His first book: a 28-day exercise plan for Yoga beginners. It's so successful that it will see new editions for the next half century. Workman also invents the desk calendar with 365 tear-off pages per year. 366 pages, some years. He launches a book of cartoons for cat lovers and calls it *Cat* – and when it doesn't sell so well, he has cat mugs made and cat pillows and cat calendars, and he sends his staff, these trinkets, and copies of *Cat* to the New York Cat Show at Madison Square Garden. In 1983 he will publish *What to Expect When You're Expecting*, and it will sell 15 million copies. When the new millenium dawns, only seven percent of America's pregnant women will say they haven't read that book.[66]

Now Workman has come across another promising book idea. Very promising, in fact. Maybe more promising than all the book ideas before. For sure: Many Americans get pregnant or might get pregnant at some point or know a pregnant American or might be directly or indirectly involved in a fellow American's pregnancy. And many Americans have cats or know cats. Or they're thinking about starting yoga. But that's nothing in comparison to breathing. It's safe to say that everyone's breathing. Those who aren't don't buy books. And there's a woman Workman has met. She's a breathing expert, without a doubt. In the not so distant future she'll point out in her book's acknowledgements section that he, Peter Workman, tempted her to write.

4. The List of Jewish Gymnastics Instructors

The year 1933 begins. Carola now has a new address and a new name and a nine-year old child. Her clients can find her in Carmerstraße, a few minutes from Zoo Station. She has married the friendly Czech, in November 1932. They spent their honeymoon in Paris. Now her name is Carola Spitz. She adopted her husband's daughter. Their apartment is big enough for Otto, Dorothea, Carola, and a gymnastics studio.

Carola also works for Elsa Gindler, in Kurfürstenstraße. On Wednesday afternoons she teaches Gindler's courses. And she's running a Gindler group for men. She's sure that nobody's as close to Gindler as she is. There was this moment in one of the courses, in April 1929, when everyone was sitting on the floor, doing some very quiet experiment, and Gindler walked through the room, stopped next to her, and handed her an envelope. Inside Carola found the official permission to teach in Gindler's name. What a gift. Everyone knows how much care Gindler takes with these things.

The Nazis organize the first boycott of Jewish business for April 1, 1933. These measures, they claim, only serve to protest the "atrocious agitation" of the foreign press. At taxi stands, men distribute handbills. These indicate which taxi companies are owned by Jews. There are quite a few Jewish-owned shops in Carola's neighborhood. The Spitz family probably sees antisemitic messages everywhere. SA men are standing in front of shops with placards saying "Germans! Defend Yourselves! Don't Buy from Jews!"

Some observers claim that most of the non-Jewish passers-by stop to read the signs because they're curious, not because they're antisemites. Compared to what follows in Germany, this spring day seems like a minor date. Witnesses do note, however, that the boycott separates Jews from an entity constructed as non-Jewish Germany. The events identify, mark, and exclude Jews. An international expert calls the boycott "an agglomeration of anti-Jewish hate in one day." In his opinion, it's far from harmless. Then there's Erich Felix, a Jewish fruit salesman, like Carola's father was when he was a young man. SA men beat him up in front of a market hall. The first suicides follow. 32-year-old Herbert Schimek, the Jewish proprietor of a Berlin waste-paper business, shoots himself on April 3.[67]

Before the Nazi years, the German gymnastics movement was splintered. Some instructors were militaristic, others poetic, some naked, some fully clothed. There were systematic gymnasts and chaotic gymnasts, Christians, Jews, the Germanic, and the cosmopolitans. Now the movement is a coherent Nazi organization. The transformation happened very quickly.

More than half a century later, the historian Saul Friedländer will study the first months of Nazi rule. He will stress how unimportant cultural life seems in this historical situation and how strange it might appear at first glance that the new rulers turned their attention to these seemingly peripheral segments. Friedländer will show, however, that targeting theater people, writers, painters (and, even more marginally, Jewish Gymnastic instructors) was greatly symbolic. Actors and actresses had audiences, writers had readers, gymnastics teachers had students. Attacks on these figures were intended to create a "split consciousness" in non-Jewish Germans. They aimed at those who perhaps didn't agree with all the exclusionary measures, but who might have felt, reared as they were on a traditional German antisemitism, that the Jewish "influence" on German culture had indeed been too extensive.[68]

In June 1933, a national gymnastics congress takes place. In a hotel on Potsdamer Platz, the participants rise to their feet and sing the Nazi hymn "Horst Wessel Lied." The Berlin gymnastics instructors all stay seated. They don't raise their hands for the Hitler salute. This may or may not be true. It's how one of them will recall events after the end of the dictatorship.[69]

Gymnastics experts are now expected to teach Germans how to function in mass rallies. The new leader of the National Gymnastics Association, a member of the Nazi Party since 1922, is convinced that only "racially unreproachable" individuals can conduct gymnastics properly. The most important German bodywork journal will soon run extensive guidelines for marches. Diagrams propose patterns: from line A to line F 2 to the center ("M") and then to line C.[70] The Nazi ideologues aim to get rid of the individual, wanting to see it dilute into the body of the "Volk," which they see as "pure" and homogenous, a "community of blood."[71]

Much later, members of the gymnastics movement will point out that the new rulers forced them to join their system. Historians will show, however, how quickly many gymnasts turned to the new regime. There was something about the premodern, irrational aspects of National Socialism that body and breathing experts may have found attractive.[72]

In the early summer of 1933 Jewish gymnastics teachers are barred from taking on non-Jewish students. In Berlin a list circulates with the names of these instructors, sorted by districts. The list provides their names and methods. Some represent the "Anna Hermann" method, some are "Mensendieck-Hirschler" teachers, some "Kallmeyer-Lauterbach," some "Gindler." There's one Lotte Kristeller on the list. She is a Gindler teacher who will one day resume her work in Tel Aviv and welcome a student named Moshé Feldenkrais to one of her classes.[73] "C. Spitz" appears as a teacher of two methods: Anna Hermann and Elsa Gindler.

The list shows 61 names. Even before 1933 there were too many gymnastics instructors competing for not enough students. Now that Jewish experts can only take on Jewish clients, their professional situation is hopeless, and the situation of non-Jewish gymnastics instructors so much better than before.[74]

In the fall of 1933, Carola Spitz is pregnant. She has a miscarriage in December. A woman named Julchen, maybe a friend, maybe a maid, is standing next to her bed when the miscarriage begins. Julchen gives Carola a flower when she leaves and says she's never seen Carola that way. So agitated. When she's feeling a bit better, Carola talks to Gindler about what happened. Gindler says the only way to get past it would be to give birth to a healthy child. That is never going to happen.

Antisemitic agitation, organized by the Nazi press, intensifies in 1935. In Munich, men smash the shop windows of Jewish businesses. They attack the shopkeepers, their customers, their staff. Many smaller German cities now make it illegal for Jews to enter movie theaters. Around the corner from Carola, Otto, and Dorothea, on Kurfürstendamm, Nazi citizens threaten Jewish passers-by. They announce "the cleansing of Berlin." They hit Jewish women in the face. Jewish men show courage. "Nobody came to their help," an observer notes.[75]

The Spitz family decide to move away from the central business district to the quiet neighborhood of Wilmersdorf. Carola has her own studio there, too, but almost no students. They send Dorothea to a Swiss boarding school, wanting to protect her from what's going on in Berlin.

In that time, Carola keeps a journal and observes how unclear the conversations with Otto are. They're always repeating things. They constantly need to ask each other follow-up questions. When they're talking, Carola's always already thinking about something else, like the next phone call she has to make. Then she isn't mindful of what she says, and surprised that Otto isn't mindful either.

Carola reflects these details of everyday life in typed reports for Elsa Gindler. She wants to solve specific problems. Where does she feel her breathing today? How does breathing out work? But she can't really explore these questions, because so many "chains of thought" are running through her head. One thing she knows: "I can't postpone starting my work to the moment when everything in life is rosy. That's impossible."

In January 1936 a Gindler course explores these issues. They talk about movement. About creeping, for instance. How could you creep like an earthworm and avoid *becoming* an earthworm? A dog can do that. Dogs crawl, which is almost the same as creeping, but dogs aren't worms, someone points out. Next they talk about lifting. How if you're lifting a heavy load, you can either turn into a "victim" of that load or remain a "non-victim." Gindler cites a student who said: "Carola in the course and Carola in life are two different things." Carola agrees.

In the fall of the year 1936 she's sitting in Gindler's course "Breathing for Beginners." She's taking notes. Breaching the new laws, non-Jewish Elsa Gindler is apparently employing Jewish Carola Spitz as her assistant. It seems to be part of Carola's job description to write long, detailed course reports.

In "Breathing for Beginners," the question of the ideal comes up. There are clients who can't deal with the fact that breathing changes. They can't accept that it's not always deep and regular. It can be shallow, choppy, depending on the circumstances. One client wonders why you sometimes feel the breath way up in your chest and sometimes deep down in your belly. These really are beginner's questions. Gindler says to just explore the movements that your breathing depends on. In your head. In your chest. In your entire body.

In one course session, two students arrive late. Very late. An entire hour. Gindler talks about being present. How in life you're usually doing something and yet you're not really there because you're thinking about something else. And that you should be conscious of that. It's important, Gindler says, to be present in the moment. It's just as important, though, to let go of perfectionist ideals.

There's this dancer in Berlin called Jutta Klamt who knows so much about breathing and about the inner strength of a person who's being herself and isn't content to just fit in. Klamt has ideals. And she's writing about them at a time when the Nazi dictatorship is already in its fourth year, and uniformity and subordination are everywhere.

Jutta Klamt posits that people who are short of breath don't have opinions. They can't think for themselves. They're opportunists. Only those who feel the breath as a "living power" within them can see the true size of life. They see "clarity," Klamt says. They see "calm." And because they're breathing the right way, they shape their character, and they turn into "upstanding people."

The author of such fascinating lines is a fervent Nazi and runs a highly successful gymnastics school in Berlin. Joseph Goebbels' children take Jutta Klamt's classes. And every lesson at her school begins and ends with mindful breathing.[76]

Carola Spitz runs a less successful institute. In the fall of 1936, though, she has three clients and meets them every Monday night, for five consecutive weeks. Carola asks these women to write about themselves.

Ellen Katz, 23 years old, doesn't write much, though enough to see that it's a typical Jewish biography of the time: Ellen quit school before graduating, probably for financial reasons, and now she's an apprentice in her father's company. She took time off for a home economics course. Now she knows how to cook and sew, wash, and iron. These are useful things if you're thinking about escaping to another country. Why she's taking a course with Carola: Ellen doesn't say.

Anni Philipson writes a bit more. She's 25. She loves skiing and rowing and tennis. She also works in her father's company, a haberdashery. She's done Gindler work before and found that it gave her so much, "emotionally, not rationally," and that it was very different from other forms of gymnastics. Looking for a teacher, it "had to be a Gindler disciple," she writes, and it had to be someone she found personally pleasing. Carola.

The oldest student, Flora Türkel, 50, composes the most detailed report. She sketches her childhood. She writes about her parents' unhappy marriage, her mother's early death, her own marriage when she was just nineteen, her husband's suicide, her move to Berlin, how inflation ruined her, how she then worked as her brother's housekeeper.

Flora Türkel wants to find the meaning of life. Her brother, she says, always made fun of her search for the intuitive, emotional side of things. Now that brother lives in California. To Flora Türkel, his departure – and that of so many others – was "soul-shattering." She feels drawn to a "more natural and simpler way of life." She wants to get rid of the "primacy of the intellect." She's hoping for "inner harmony" and the "dissolution" of the "condition of fear" that has taken a hold of her body.

In the studio Carola asks the three women to stand. Just stand. She wants them to notice their bodies. She wants them to realize how being cramped up or being too limp are obstacles to any form of activity. She wants them to know that being calm for a while isn't some sort of stagnation. You could see it as a phase of regeneration. She wants to show them that saying something like "I can't bend down because of my back" can't be true if you don't even notice your back. It's about feeling it. They discuss whether people must fall victim to situations or whether there may not be options to get out of passivity.

Flora Türkel is never going to make it to California. She will be murdered at the Sobibor death camp.[77] In the Berlin studio she asks Carola what's going to happen once she starts to feel. Is it going to change anything? Carola says that only practical experiments will deliver the answer. In one of the next sessions, Ellen, Anni, and Flora all stand with one foot on a gymnastics cudgel. Now the body will notice something. The body, not the head. She has her students look at each other. She asks them to practice looking.

Carola gets the three students to lie down on broomsticks. When Flora Türkel feels the stick beneath her, she notices how her body adapts. Her circulation is so much stronger now. When she gets up, she feels as if she'd just gotten a massage. And after the course is over, Flora hands in a long, enthusiastic report. In Carola's studio, for the very first time, she really felt her body. Flora writes that it all makes perfect sense to her now.

In the spring of 1937, Carola reaches for a pile of old stationery. They show her old letterhead, the one advertising the studio in Offenbacher Straße, the place she gave up because she got married.

On the back of these pages, she writes her life story. Visiting the Olympic Games, twice, in the summer of 1936. Passing a swimming test in September 1921. How she felt like a cripple as a child because she always had trouble with her neck. How her brother hit her with toys. How she remembers being on her father's arm "in the glow of the Christmas tree" and how her brother took his toy tomahawk, she calls it an "Indian axe," and hit her eye so she almost went blind. And how it still felt so horrible to listen to her brother scream when he was beaten by their parents.

When she's in her eighties, she will describe her mother and father as sophisticated cosmopolitans, shining examples to her. In these pages, in 1937, a different picture emerges. Her father she sketches as selfish, her mother as a "forever serious, frugal woman." To note that "Mutti is laughing," she says, had been an exceptional observation. She'll later reach for a pencil to add that her mother was very interested in "intellectual problems." That sounds a bit more positive. She tells the story of how she, Carola, discovered gymnastics, her years with Anna Hermann, the change to Elsa Gindler's circle, her marriage, and her sudden motherhood. She's been married for more than four years now and she still hasn't found a way to balance "professional issues and family demands."

Carola has plenty more sheets of letterheaded paper. Nobody needs the stationery of a studio that no longer exists. She could go on writing. She could discuss her life between 1933 and 1937. But she adds just two more sentences. "Then again, due to the political events, the time wasn't suited to provide the necessary quiet to solve personal questions." She crosses out "questions" and replaces the term with "conflicts." Then she notes, three and a half years after the event, her miscarriage, from which, she says, she found it very hard to recover. That's how her story ends.

August Glucker says: "Breathing is life." He's a 1930s gymnastics teacher who has profited from this new era. When his voice sounds from the radio in the morning, people say: "Es gluckert." In other words: it's gluckering. From the studio Glucker greets his "dear morning gymnasts" and takes them through some exercises. When he's not behind the microphone, he writes guidebooks, for the more passionate devotees of gluckering. *Fresh and Free!* he dedicates to women, *Strong and Happy!* to men. Women, Glucker says, should be "at the frontline of physical exercise." It's their responsibility to bring forth a "healthy and strong race." Glucker shows that there's a wrong way to do domestic dusting (pelvis tilted too far back) and a right way (body erect). There's also a right and wrong way to carry things. And there's a wrong way of breathing: overly weak and rushed. The correct form of inhaling, Glucker says, depends on power:

powerful lungs, powerful breathing muscles, and the powerful movement of the diaphragm.[78]

One day the Nazis will take Otto to prison and that will change everything. In the preceding years, Carola and Otto keep returning to Berlin. From Znaim and Brno in Czechoslovakia, in the spring of 1934. From Rome and Capri and Florence half a year later. In 1935 they return from Palestine, where they had explored business opportunities for Otto. They come back from Znaim and Prague in January 1936. From London in March 1936, in July 1936 from Venice and Bolzano, and a year later from the island of Rab, Yugoslavia.

Maybe they feel safe in Berlin because of Otto's Czech passport. Maybe he doesn't have any significant business problems there. His factory doesn't have store windows that antisemitic slogans could be painted on. His cigarettes, though, coming from a Jewish factory, could be refused by shopkeepers loyal to antisemitic principles. Then there's the Nazi campaign against smoking. Tobacco is now declared an enemy of the people. Germany is fighting "tobacco terror" and "tobacco capitalism."[79] And yet, none of this seems to affect Otto's business. There are times, in fact, when the factory struggles to keep up with the demand and Carola must help out. The future author of *Breathing: The ABCs* drives around Berlin, stops at shops, jumps out of the car, and delivers cartons of Kraj Orient, Prima, Luxus, Club, and Cabinet.

Maybe Otto remains successful because he's found a niche: his special brand, the so-called "Russian" cigarettes. And maybe, he's in his late forties now, he can't imagine starting anew in another country. The same might be true of Carola. Her career has slowed down so much that she might not feel ready for a new beginning. And maybe they don't think of leaving because they live in Berlin. German Jews feel safe here. Lots of Jews are leaving Germany's small towns now; they're moving to the big, anonymous city because they think it's more secure. Otto and Carola already live where these migrants are heading.[80]

In September 1937 they are visiting Thea in Switzerland when Carola's mother calls them from Berlin. She says that someone must have entered their apartment. Several men. Maybe the Gestapo. And that these men forced her to accompany them to the bank and open Otto's safe deposit. Let's not go back to Germany, Carola says. We're going back, says Otto. They're back in Berlin when the doorbell rings. Much later Carola will recall two Gestapo men and a regular policeman, standing in their living room, looking at the bookshelves. Pestalozzi, the Gestapo man says. That sounds foreign. Pestalozzi's an 18th century Swiss philosopher and, to Germans, not so outrageously "foreign." But she doesn't say anything. The regular policeman then points at the red volumes of Goethe's collected works. Goethe, he says. He's very German. The Gestapo men don't respond. They take Otto with them. The policeman hangs back a few steps when they leave. On the doorstep, he turns to Carola. Under his breath he says: If he's not back by five, he won't be back at all.

There's this thing called the "Surén-Schurz." It's a loincloth that doesn't leave much to the imagination. When its inventor Hans Surén displays his body for the camera, he uses large amounts of oil for the parts not covered by the "Schurz."

Like radio gymnast August Glucker, Hans Surén has adapted perfectly to the new political developments. His hands press on his shiny chest, his thumbs rest on his nipples. He demonstrates the proper method of "chest breathing." He stands on tip-toes and raises his arms up high. He calls this: "Big breathing in taut execution." He demonstrates what people should do with an iron ball. Throw the ball and breathe out. Catch the ball and breathe in. Women are photographed doing Surén's exercises. They're not even wearing a "Schurz." Surén says that men should breathe with their bellies and use flank and chest breathing when they're doing something physically demanding. Women, he says, should always use chest breathing. He points out that among gorillas, the differences in breathing are also gendered.

Surén's book *Breathing Gymnastics* emerges as a 1930s bestseller. His other titles are also extremely popular. There's *The Man and the Sun*, his treatise on nudism, and his guidebook *Massaging Yourself*. Surén's *Breathing Gymnastics* are taught in courses run by Nazi youth organizations, by the SA and SS. His writings are part of an official ideology constantly revolving around the body: the body of the "Volk," the "Aryan body," the body of the "pure race." There's always another body contrasted with that concept: the imperfect, foreign body, which, according to this new German ideology, will have to be expulsed.[81]

Otto Spitz doesn't come back at five. He's in a prison on Alexanderplatz. Nobody knows why. Maybe Carola thinks that they'll let him go the next day. That doesn't happen. Days go by, weeks go by. Every day, Carola goes to Alexanderplatz. There's a limit on visits. Nobody gets to visit every day. The officer in charge of visits has a ledger in front of him. He asks her whether she keeps a record of her visits. No, she says. He says: I don't either. Carola keeps visiting every day. Whenever she's feeling scared, she thinks of Gindler's work. She wants to act. Not be a victim.

Fig. 7: Otto Spitz's cigarette factory.

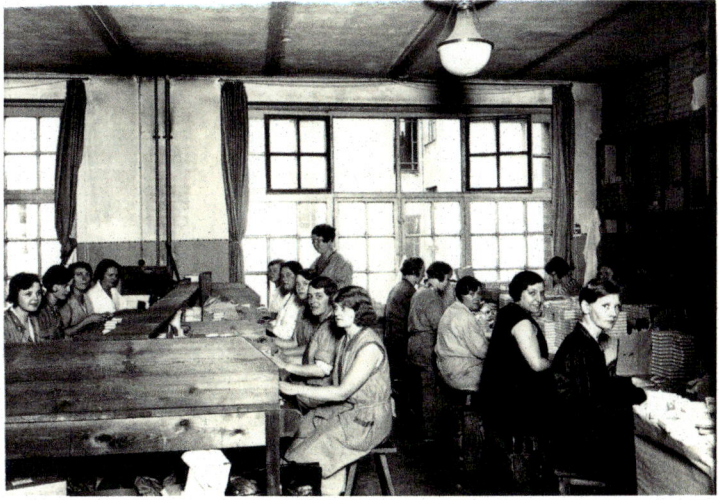

Otto is a man who just can't be by himself. And now he's in solitary confinement. Then they put him in a cell with a few Jehovah's Witnesses, people who refuse to say "Heil Hitler," because they only salute God. They share their food with him, they show him how to make the bed and how not to get in trouble. Once Carola manages to have Otto freed for a few hours. He's needed in the cigarette factory, she says. He'll have to mix the different kinds of tobacco, and only he knows the special recipes. Policemen accompany Otto and Carola to the factory. Otto offers them some of his purest tobacco. They smoke, they cough, they gasp, and ask whether he's trying to poison them. And yet they let him go home, too, the same day, for a brief visit. One policeman comes along. Carola fixes some sandwiches for Otto and asks whether the officer would also like one. He says they don't allow him to accept food in Jewish households. Then he takes Otto back to prison. Otto is a Jew in German captivity, late in the year 1937.

1938 begins. The weeks of imprisonment have turned into months. Carola and her lawyer Richard Auerbach are on their way to Hotel Adlon. She's supposed to meet an American who might be able to help. At the hotel, she hands money over to him. A lot of money. She asks what he's going to do with it. The American says that he might discuss cases with his contacts and then the binder containing the case might appear on the desk and then the contact might need to go to the bathroom and then he might leave the money in the binder. He just wanted to meet her to make sure he would recognize her voice. She goes back to the apartment. She waits for his call. At midnight, the phone rings. She picks up and says her name. It's the American. All he says is: You will need to see the ambassador.

She makes an appointment in the Czech embassy. She enters the giant office and looks at the long narrow carpet running diagonally across the room. It ends right before His Excellency Vojtěch Mastný's desk. She approaches the desk, across the carpet, and she's still several steps away when she notices that His Excellency is cross-eyed. Here he is, as important as the Emperor of China, she thinks, and this is what he looks like.

Mastný asks her a few questions. Then he says he's about to send a démarche. She doesn't know what that is. It's the last measure taken before there's war, he says. She looks at him, confused. There's not going to be war, he says. Of course not. It's just a démarche. He's sure they'll free her

4. The List of Jewish Gymnastics Instructors

husband soon. And once they do, they should both leave Germany within 48 hours. His Excellency walks her along the carpet to the door and then asks in a very low voice how much she paid her contact. She tells him. He thanks her.

It's midnight again when the American calls to tell her that they're going to release Otto. In the morning a policeman calls to tell her the same thing. She says: I know. She shouldn't have said that. How did she know? The policeman's curious. She says the embassy had called.

Otto gets out of prison, nonetheless. She wants to leave Berlin and Germany right away. He wants to go back to the factory one last time. So they go. They take a tour. The men and women working the machines are looking at Otto. The women filling the cigarette boxes are looking at Otto. Nobody says anything. In his office Otto asks one of his staff why they were all so quiet. The man says they had practiced a song to sing for him, a song to welcome him back. But then, when they saw him, they couldn't sing. He's gotten so thin during his months in prison. They just couldn't sing.

On a Monday night, February 21, 1938, they take two suitcases and board a train to Prague. Once they've passed the German-Czech border, they both fall asleep. For the time being, they're staying in Prague. Otto's relatives feed them. One meal follows the next, for days on end. Otto needs that. Then they move on to Italy, to Ospedaletti on the Mediterranean. From there they go to Amsterdam. Dorothea arrives. They've taken her out of the Swiss boarding school. They want her to be with them. Otto's mother Rudolfina also joins them. A few weeks later, she dies in a Dutch hospital.

Otto's trying to start cigarette production in Amsterdam, to no avail. In Germany a company named "Phänomen" takes over his tobacco, his machines, his client register, and the staff of "Kraj." They're paying zero Reichsmark for this. The new owners send letters to Otto's customers and introduce themselves as "Aryan" cigarette makers. Otto, Carola, and Dorothea apply for U.S. immigration visas. They may have to wait a very long time. It seems certain that they've waited too long to apply.

In the summer of 1938 Carola asks former clients for letters of recommendation. A gynecologist writes wonderful lines. Ernst Solms says that Carola's gymnastics made him so much stronger: his body, his breathing, and therefore his "soul." And Carola, he says, was such a fantastic person. Solms will survive the war by going into hiding in the Netherlands.[82]

The chemist Alfred Schnell will go underground in the same country. He will be denounced and shot.[83] His letter says that Carola's courses were such an "excellently effective counterbalance to working a desk job." His "vitality" had intensified because of her. Schnell writes that she taught him "to better adapt to complicated situations in everyday life, and to develop a better sense for them."

Mali Goldschmidt testifies that she learned from Carola Spitz to "adapt her body to the most difficult conditions." Carola had opened her up to "how unbelievably important it was to know more about the function of the muscles and the respiratory organs." Mali Goldschmidt feels "infinite regret" not to be able to continue with Carola's courses. She lives in Palestine now. She adds a private letter to her official recommendation and advises Carola to go to New York. There's this other Berlin gymnastics teacher, one of Mali's cousins, Elsa Henschke, and she opened a "fantastic studio" there, Mali writes. People are saying, Mali reports, that she's one of the best gymnastics teachers in all of New York. Mali believes, off the record, that Carola is "so much better than Elsa H."

Their visa numbers don't come up. Nobody knows how long they'll have to wait. Otto thinks France will be safer than the small Netherlands, should the Nazis decide to attack. And they've heard that in Paris you can do more to speed up the visa waiting period. In October 1938 they receive papers for France. They move, the three of them.

Carola's mother Paula is still living in Berlin. She takes care of all kinds of errands for Carola and Otto. At Zoo Station she posts suitcases for them. The suitcases take the train and arrive, unopened, in Paris. Paula supervises the removal of furniture and household objects from the Berlin apartment. In an overseas container all this will be shipped to New York. If everything goes to plan, Carola and Otto and Dorothea will follow the container. And after that, they will bring Carola's mother over. Of course they will.

When Carola, Otto, and Dorothea Spitz arrive in Paris, German refugees aren't particularly well regarded. In December 1937 a German killed several people in the metropolitan region. Parisians remember that.[84] And France in general has a refugee problem. That's how people see it: You can't let them all in. Only very few Germans are granted work permits. Most of them sink into poverty. There are suicides. There are stories of refugees starving to death in their Parisian hotel rooms.[85] Now, after the November 1938 pogroms across Germany, even more migrants will arrive.

There was a conference at Evian in July 1938. It could have solved the refugee crisis. Representatives of thirty-two nations convened. There were half a million people to be distributed. No government made any reliable offers, except for the dictator of the Dominican Republic. In Germany the Nazi press expressed antisemitic delight: It seemed as though Jews weren't welcome anywhere.[86]

In Paris the Spitzs live first in a hotel, then in an apartment, then another hotel, then another apartment. They keep waiting for their visas. They constantly have to ask for new French papers. It's impossible to truly be sure they'll ever make it to the United States. Carola and Otto have sold their bonds. They can still live. They're privileged. But war might break out any day now.

The three of them live together, in Ville d'Avray. Otto had to give up what he loved most in life: his cigarette factory. Dorothea is a postadolescent girl who was so extraordinarily happy in her Swiss boarding school in Hasliberg and then had to leave. And Carola only feels whole when she's teaching mindfulness and just can't teach anymore.

In Washington, D.C., the Chairman of the Committee for Un-American Activities reminds his colleagues to ignore sentimental, immigration-friendly appeals. He proposes to close the gates to America and then throw the keys away. No United States consulate will want to be known as lenient in dispensing visas. The Parisian office is no exception. The zeitgeist matters. In April 1939, eighty-three percent of Americans say they're opposed to higher immigrant quotas. Lawmakers discuss humanitarian measures – letting in refugee children, for instance. An influential politician's wife points out that 20,000 beautiful children will eventually turn into 20,000 "ugly adults."[87]

In May 1939 Otto Spitz is drifting around Paris. They can't just keep waiting. He visits agencies selling expensive, though dubious, visa options to other countries. It's not the first time he's making these rounds. Then he writes to a former colleague at the cigarette factory: Sigismund Sternson, Berlin. Sternson's desperate. He must get out. Otto, one step ahead, suggests Bolivia, Cuba, maybe England.

Two and a half weeks later Otto hears that Sternson's going to take a train to Naples and then a ship to Shanghai. Jewish migrants don't need visas there. Now Sternson seems saved, and the fate of the family Spitz remains undecided. Otto sends Sternson his best. Not long after, he will learn that Sternson has started to produce cigarettes in Shanghai, just like in the good old days.

In August 1939 they're still in Paris. Still no visas. Mali gets in touch from Palestine. She empathizes with Carola, sends advice, encourages her. Carola is so "stable, so solid," Mali says. She sends a picture of herself, her husband and two donkeys transporting "chicken manure." She reports on the plum harvest, the peach harvest, the tomato harvest. It's hot in Palestine and sometimes, working in the gardens, Mali thinks about Carola: how she would have told her to loosen up the body and not to invest too much force. Mali now advises against going to the United States. People are saying that there might be a dramatic turn to antisemitism in America as well.

When World War II breaks out, they still don't have visas. There is no indication whatsoever that Gindler work, conscious breathing, or any other mindfulness techniques make Carola's life any easier at that time. In Paris the authorities intern all German and Austrian men aged between 17 and 56. It's supposed to last a few days. Then it takes weeks. Otto is a Czech national. They don't intern him.[88]

Autumn comes, winter, and spring. And then, on April 1, 1940, Carola Spitz, listed as a German citizen, receives visa number 25719 from the United States consulate. Otto holds visa number 1060, for Czech nationals, and Dorothea, also Czech, number 1061.

Carola's mother has made it to Amsterdam by now. She tells them how happy she is for them. She asks her granddaughter to keep a diary for her about the Atlantic crossing. Then again, Paula Joseph notes, Dorothea might be too seasick to write. She also asks what to do with the jacket she's been knitting for Dorothea. It's only half done.

Otto, Carola, and Thea have three tickets for a passage on May 19, 1940. That's six weeks away. Once again, they're waiting. Every day brings frightening news. On May 10, German troops occupy the Netherlands, Belgium, and Luxemburg. On May 15 the Netherlands capitulate. On May 17 the Germans occupy Brussels. From there it's just another 300 kilometers to Paris. On May 18, 1940, their passports receive their final European stamps in Sainte-Nazaire, the harbor close to Nantes, south of Brittany. On Sunday, May 18, German troops reach Northern France.

Decades later, in 1991, Carola will tell her grandson Steven about the passage, and Steven is going to take notes. They had first-class tickets, she tells him, though records say they travelled in third. She will say that most of the time she slept in one of those wicker chairs. That they played a good deal of table tennis to pass the time. "GERMANS IN PARIS:" That was the headline they saw on the pier, in New York. Which is unlikely. They reached the city on May 27 and the Germans occupied Paris on June 14. Maybe all these events cluster together in her memory: their rescue becoming even more dramatic, in first class, on the last ship out, into New York harbor, where Otto, and this could be true, of course, bought lots of sandwiches and passed them around to all sorts of people who happened to be passing by on the pier. One thing is definitely accurate: The S.S. Champlain, which saved the lives of Otto, Carola, and Dorothea Spitz, and, on the same journey, the lives of Vera and Vladimir Nabokov, will hit a German mine only three weeks later and sink.[89]

They move on to Cleveland, Ohio, and then, very quickly, back to New York. They find an apartment in Washington Heights. They can see Broadway from the back windows and a schoolyard from the front of the apartment. Just a few blocks away are the Hudson River and George Washington Bridge.

They are living in a parallel society. More than 20,000 German Jewish refugees have moved to Washington Heights since 1933. German is spoken in homes and on the streets. These people aren't Berlin intellectuals. Most of them come from towns and cities in southern or western Germany. Many of them are far more religious than the Spitz family, though that isn't saying much. The new arrivals establish a dozen synagogues. There are numerous kosher German butchers and an organization for "Immigrant Jewish War Veterans" – veterans of World War One, on the German side. Some people call this neighborhood the "Fourth Reich." Some New York Jews find it utterly embarrassing that the new inhabitants of Washington Heights speak German when they're standing on street corners.[90]

Carola notices the dark dust on the windows. The air in New York is extremely polluted. She's impressed by the coin-operated washing machines in the basement. She sends her mother registered packages. Bright pink slips come back to her, signed by Paula Joseph in Amsterdam.

Carola wants to do everything she can to get her mother here. They own $ 12,571.40. This is the amount they cite on the "Affidavit of Support" for her mother's U.S. visa application. Carola writes letters to the State Department in Washington and to the American Consulate in Rotterdam. She certifies that Paula Joseph will not become a burden to anyone. She, Carola Spitz, will always take care of her. It is her explicit desire, she writes, to make the last years of her mother's life "as wonderful as I can."

Her mother, Paula Joseph, 73 years old, now lives in Vossiusstraat, Amsterdam, on Vondelpark, a few blocks away from the Rijksmuseum, in a small boarding house run by the Meyers. Paula tells Carola, Otto, and Dorothea: "We don't have to believe in seeing each other again. I won't live to see that day." She writes that she will come to terms with her "useless life" ending in Amsterdam. She is "jobless" during the day and "sleepless" at night. She walks along the Amstel. She takes walks in the park. She finds the park "wonderful." Her landlords, she says, mean well. Again and again, she writes how healthy she is. From time to time the Meyers add notes to Paula's letters, saying they're not to worry. They will take care of Carola's mother.

In their American apartment, 660 Fort Washington Avenue, they have German chairs, tables, wardrobes, and beds. The container with Otto's and Carola's furniture had been waiting for them since March 1939. The record collection stayed behind in Berlin, but the record player is in New York. Their German-Persian rugs cover the New York floors. The Limoges service has arrived safe and sound, the glasses, and the other china. And there's a medicine ball on this side of the Atlantic, and a rubber ball, five jumping ropes, six gymnastics cudgels.

It's September 1940, a cold September, and in Amsterdam, Paula Joseph is freezing. Coal is rationed. Fall hasn't even begun and she's already wearing her wool jacket and her warmest underwear. From time to time, she sees the Meyers for tea, but tea is also rationed. She is gloomy because she has nothing to do. In her room there's no space and no air. All the boarding house laundry is hung up to dry in her room. She goes for walks in the streets, through the park. She observes how the seasons change the park. For her 74th birthday, she receives visitors who bring chocolate, flowers, fruit. She buys some cake for her fellow tenants and writes a poem for the small party. To her daughter she writes that her poetry "can't compete" with "her predecessor Goethe." She assumes that her granddaughter is collecting postal stamps in New York. "Strength is growing along with the worries," Paula Joseph says. She's getting older and lonelier, but she's also becoming more independent. She says these years are like living the last years of her youth once again. For now, it's still possible to emigrate from Germany, but you can't get out of the Netherlands anymore. Her real birthday wish, she writes, "is to wander off into the hereafter quickly, abruptly, and without prior illness."

Around that time Carola takes on her first job in New York. She writes to her mother about the first 28 dollars she has made. She has one student. It's a start. She reaches out to her friends from the Berlin years, Otto Fenichel, his wife Claire. The Fenichels knows a psychoanalyst in a hospital run by Yale University. Carola finds a client there. It's a long commute, but it's the next step. She takes the train from Grand Central to New Haven, Connecticut, teaches relaxation, gets on the train back to the city. Then she takes on another student. Liesel Edelmuth. Liesel's husband, Fritz, a German chemist, has found a job in New Haven. Obviously the Edelmuths have made it in the United States. Carola and Otto haven't.

In Amsterdam Paula Joseph is delighted to hear that her granddaughter is attending school in New York City. She hopes to "celebrate her achievements" sometime in the future. She advises Thea to work particularly hard in American history and she mentions President Lincoln and hopes that Dorothea will remember his words about equality and the love between human beings. Paula's letters look different now. The paper is thin, her handwriting very small. She crams as many words as possible onto the pages.

In the boarding house in Vossiusstraat, the male tenants play bridge a lot. The duvet's keeping Paula Joseph warm in bed, though not always. In January 1941 she's freezing cold and in pain. She visits the committee for Jewish emigration and talks to a "very likable, nice, matter-of-fact gentleman" who says he's going to take on her case. He promises to do everything he can. There's talk about a visa option for aged parents of recent immigrants. Paula Joseph learns that all hotels in Amsterdam are now closed to Jews. So are the restaurants. It is the second time she's witnessing this process. First in Berlin, now here. "Always something new," she writes. In February 1941 she's watching people skate on the canals. The mood among the refugees, Paula Joseph notes, is "gloomy, expectant, and hopeful."

The movie theaters of Amsterdam close to Jews, and so do the cafés. Carola's brother Heinz has left Gurs camp in the Southwest of France. He's now in a different camp and works in an auto shop. Paula admonishes her family in New York for being too extravagant with express mail and telegrams. "Everything will be fine," she writes. Then she finally, officially, receives a slot for leaving Europe. She's booked on HMS Exeter. Departure from Lisbon: September 5, 1941.

People in Amsterdam don't meet for tea anymore. Paula doesn't believe that her crossing will take place. "So I'll wait for the end of the war," she writes, "or for my death." She says: "If one doesn't happen, the other will." She has to change her dresses, because she's doesn't have enough to eat.

Paula reads a lot. A nonfiction book she's reading, Anton Zischka's *Bread for Two Billion People*, tells the story of hunger and how people have always struggled for bread, for space, for a dignified life. Zischka concludes that humankind has finally learned one thing: "to live without killing."[91] In August 1941 Paula Joseph learns that she has lost her place on the Exeter. American passengers are preferred. "Somehow you push through, by and by, and you get tougher and tougher," she says. Because she's Jewish, she now has to walk around the park.

From New York her daughter reports on some problems she has with her gallbladder and that she can't eat pickles. Paula Joseph advises her on the gallbladder issues. She also tells her that two very thin slices of pickles on a slice of bread thinly spread with butter is what constitutes lunch for her in Amsterdam. She writes: "I'd love to be able to say that I can't eat pickles." Carola sends her the new stationery for her relaxation studio in Manhattan and Paula Joseph finds complimentary words.

Carola and Otto are reading *Aufbau*. The paper runs an ad for a show called *Das Weisse Rössl am Central Park*, at Cafe Vienna on 77th Street. It's billed as a musical "in bad German, and English that's just as bad." *Aufbau* readers learn that "internationally known stars" are performing in a place called Old Europe on Broadway, that the Fred Le Quorne Dance Studios are teaching dance courses of the Fred Le Quorne Method, and that the Louise Schwarz Culinary School offers one-on-one lessons in making "fancy sandwiches."

On the back pages of the paper, an author named Hannah Arendt explores Jewish identity in the era of forced mass migration. To Arendt the "refugees chased from country to country" are "the avantgarde of their peoples." The 19th century knew "global citizens," Arendt writes. Now there's a new type: "involuntary global travelers." These travelers, Arendt points out, will have to be conscious of their own political significance in order to fight for the freedom of the Jewish people.

Aufbau also reports from Europe. Four hundred young Dutch Jews have died in Mauthausen camp, from malnutrition and brutal forced labor. Escaping persecution has once again become more difficult. There are no trains from Germany to Lisbon anymore. This *Aufbau* issue notes that the Nazis are apparently working on "a different system to 'solve the Jewish question.'" [92]

From Amsterdam, in these November days, Paula Joseph writes her final long letter to her daughter, son-in-law and granddaughter. After that, she will only be able to send a few lines via the Red Cross. Once again, she tells them that she's in good health. She's spending more time with the Meyers now, partly because of the "warmth of socializing," partly because of "the warmth of their rooms." From time to time she has small gifts for their fellow tenants, so "she's someone" in the boarding house, she says, "a tiny someone."

She spends time in her room reading. Difficult books. Reading keeps her from other "useless" thoughts. She's 75 now. From time to time, she makes a cup of tea or coffee. Carola has managed to send her a package; Paula is making its contents last. Occasionally someone gives her a piece of zwieback, sometimes some gingerbread. The undernourished reader Paula Joseph, who continues to lose weight, writes to her daughter that she is happy to "learn about the many connections of life and the events taking place in the world."

5. Flowers from Charlotte

In her little office on Central Park West – no view of the park –, Carola is writing her book. On the wall hangs a picture of her mother. Medical handbooks sit on her desk. She wants to produce a helpful guide to breathing. But she doesn't want to pretend things are simple. She isn't Charlotte. She doesn't write about doing the dishes with a smiling heart. First she presents the theoretical foundations. She explores the stimuli that impact the breathing center of our body. Then she points out how hard it is to change routines.

There's not one correct way of breathing, she writes, only different versions of breathing that seem right for specific situations. She recommends the early morning as the ideal time for breathing experiments. You should choose a quiet place. Avoid drafts. Select a spot that's not too warm and certainly not too cold. The fewer clothes you're wearing, the more air will touch your skin. That in itself will incite breathing. Sit cross-legged, on a mat, feet bare. Breathe for five minutes or ten, or a half hour or more. Don't overdo it. Breathing is not a test of your endurance. But you will need a certain amount of patience. Carola recommends not flitting from one position to the next.

She does suggest a wide range of experiments, though. There's the one with the straws and the one involving tapping, the one with the open mouth and the one where you go "ssssss," the pressure experiments and the leaning and the bending ones, the humming, and the stretching. She provides her tips for future nonsmokers, for those short of breath, and for those who would like to lose a few pounds (when you feel a little hungry, don't go looking for a snack – do three to five minutes of straw or ssssss-breathing). For readers with headaches, she recommends grabbing a piece of skin, on the chest or back, not the stomach, and pulling that piece of skin away from the body and breathing consciously and then letting go once the breathing has deepened. And to repeat that several times. This experiment, she says, works in the same way that the loosening of a belt works. Sometimes when you have a headache, your entire body will seem to narrow. And this experiment will take care of that.

The breathing expert also turns her attention to readers who feel that their creativity is blocked. Carola Speads advises them to choose their favorite experiment and work on it until their breathing is free of all obstacles. If your breathing is unsatisfying and disturbed, you won't be productive and you won't have ideas. The lifting and pushing of heavy objects, she says, is the only activity that requires holding your breath. At the very end of her book, she cites one of her students: Breathing with her method, this person once said, made life like "a glimpse of paradise."

In November 1978 *Breathing: The ABC's* hits the book market. The debut author is 77 years old. More than half a century ago, Pössenbacher, Munich, asked her to write a book for them. 20 years ago she sent an official document to a German reparations authority stating that she would soon stop her professional activity because she was getting too old. On the cover of her book, a dark-haired young woman appears in profile, her eye make-up conspicuous, her lips slightly parted.[93] The background is dark. From the model's mouth, the title of the book appears in white lettering against a black background.

In restaurants Otto always got up from the table when he sensed that she was about to get up. He pulled her chair back for her, and then, after she'd left, he moved the chair back to the table and sat down again. He got back up when she returned, pulled her chair away from the table and pushed it gently forward as she sat down. A gentleman. As a four-year-old he'd left Znaim, the capital of the Moravian pickle business. Znaim's name has been Znojmo for a while. After his father's death he left school early to support his family. He just barely made it out of Europe. He always called her "little mouse" and held her hand when they went for walks. He dies at the age of 92, on January 20, 1980.

Fig. 8: Breathing: The ABC's

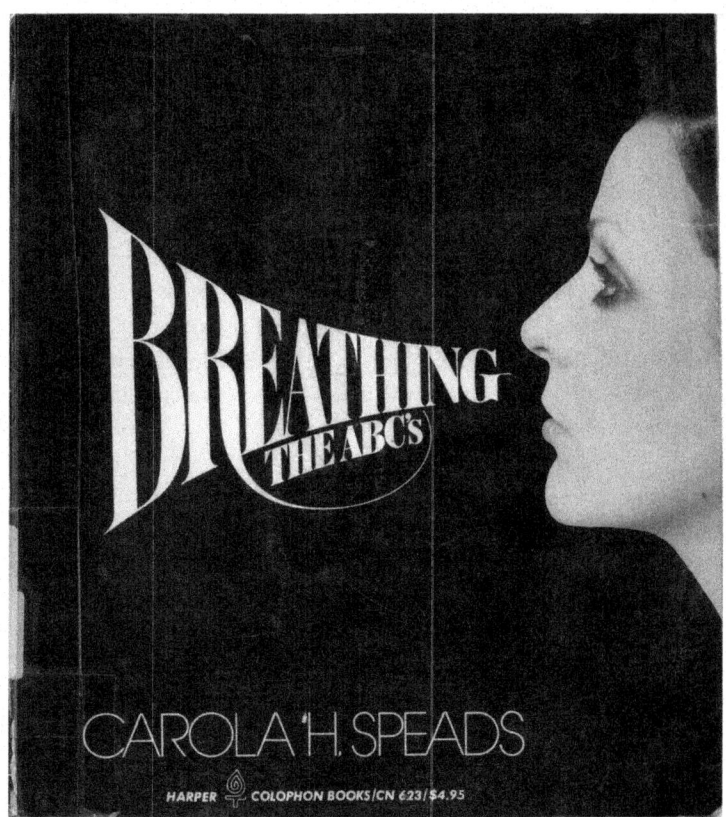

In the first phase of her grief, Carola's student Bob Chapra teaches her classes for her. Bob sits where she often sat, beneath the wall tapestry. He looks at the students. He asks them what they're feeling. They answer. He suggests an experiment. They start working. Bob feels like a mother watching her small child. He notices how the consciousness of the group seems to change as the lessons progress. What a peculiar transformation it is. It's not him. It's the group. The course seems to have a life of its own.

But then Carola comes back. Her career has only just begun. The condolences she receives after Otto's death are often also letters of congratulation on the success of her book. People praise *Breathing*. She gives interviews and tells her life story, from her first hiking tours with the Wandervögel to her work with Gindler to the methods she employs today. *Mademoiselle* turns to her for the big series "The Right Way to Do 73 Different Things." She's the expert, who else, who explains breathing to *Mademoiselle's* readers. In Amsterdam, her first city of exile, *Breathing* is published as *Ademhaling*. In Paris, her subsequent place of refuge, it's titled *ABC de la Respiration*. The Spanish edition: *ABC de la Respiración*. The German edition, *Natürliches Atmen*, doesn't have a glamourous model on the cover; it shows a tree on a meadow.[94]

However impressed readers are: Carola's book doesn't turn into a runaway success. The competition is intense. In 1978 a book about jogging dominates the nonfiction bestseller list. The author James Fixx promises that running will make your life better and longer. In 1984, at the age of 52, he will collapse and die after his daily run. But there's no telling at this point. After *The Complete Book of Running*, another very successful title takes over: *How to Flatten Your Stomach*. Soon after *Thinner Thighs in 30 Days* will sell a million copies in just six months.

Is *Breathing* too complicated? In these predigital times, Americans want books to advise them on how to reinvent themselves, or at least how to stay healthy and attractive. Or how to stay afloat financially. People believe in self-improvement and that reading will guide the way.

Half a year after *Thinner Thighs*, the follow-up volume, *30 Days to a Better Bust*, sells 360,000 copies in just four weeks.[95] And even in the segment of breathing books, Carola has formidable rivals. In 1989 Sheldon Hendler publishes *The Oxygen Breakthrough*. He claims that breathing can cure all diseases, including AIDS. A few years later author Pam Grout will guarantee that you'll lose ten pounds in just three weeks by breathing in the exact way Pam Grout suggests.[96] Carola promises that her experiments will enable her readers to see paradise. That may not be specific enough.

The Korzinskis believe in Carola. Every Sunday morning, in Hawthorne, New Jersey, they get into a Volvo and drive off to Manhattan. He's a car salesman, she's a psychotherapist. They've known each other since they were kids. They spent a lot of evenings at the "Polish Home" in Paterson, dancing the Polka and the Mazurka. Paul Korzinski used to run a towing service. After accidents on Route 208, he would go out to haul in wrecked cars. Now he owns a Volvo dealership, a make he chose because they produce the safest vehicles. When the Korzinskis drive off on Sunday mornings, they often take up to three of their four adult kids along. They cross the Hudson on the George Washington Bridge, then they take a right to the Upper West Side. It's not too complicated to find parking on the weekend, and then the four or five of them get out of the Volvo, into the elevator and go up to the tenth floor.

Paul Korzinski played football in High School and volunteered to serve in World War Two. He wanted to see the world. In Hiroshima, after the end of the war, he realized that the ashes under the soles of his boots were the remains of burned people. One day he admits to his youngest son that he always starts crying when he talks about his experiences in Japan. But he doesn't want anyone to witness that. He says he doesn't want to appear like a "fucking pussy." So he doesn't talk about these things.

In Carola's studio, Paul breathes and thinks about how that feels. He doesn't have to talk. He walks around and balances a medicine ball on his head. He breathes in, pauses, and breathes out. Carola's students don't wear swimming trunks and bathing suits anymore. They now wear white leggings and sweatshirts. On one occasion, there's a pretty big hole in Paul's leggings and this creates considerable amusement in the Studio of Physical Re-Education. He feels how much this work helps his back, which he ruined playing football, and maybe also the pain left behind by his time as a soldier.

And then, after 90 minutes in Carola's studio, all Korzinskis feel better. They change, take the elevator down, and go get bagels. The Volvo takes them back to New Jersey.

Fig. 9: Carola Speads in the studio

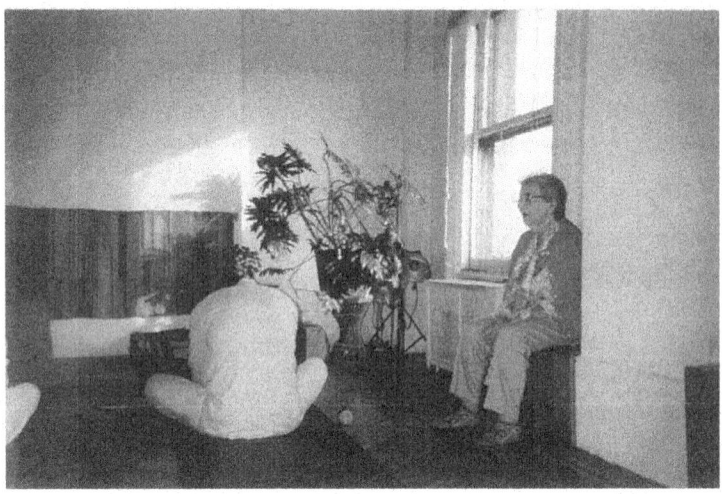

Carola's grandson Alan takes a video camera and visits her in her apartment. He turns on the camera. "Why don't you tell us about some of your things, Omi?" That's how the conversation begins. She's standing next to the glass cabinet with the china and points at tea pots. She tells Alan who these tea pots belonged to. Then she sits down, on the sofa, and talks about her grandfather in Germany who owned horses. When his favorite horse died, he had it stuffed. She tells stories about her parents and their extensive travels and how their Aunt Lieschen, who didn't have kids, looked after Heinz and Carola when they were away. Her parents went to Egypt and took a boat up the Nile, a week-long trip, and down the Nile again, another week. And then they brought a crocodile back to Berlin. The crocodile was also stuffed. She talks about her "Mademoiselle," who gave her private French lessons, and the "Miss" who taught English. The bakery on the first floor of their building was Berlin's best bakery, she says. Then Alan asks what things were like in the war and the Nazi era, and she tells him about Otto's time in prison and about everything she did until he finally got out.

Harry stops by, the husband of Frances, her niece. They live on the Upper West Side and he's a schoolteacher on the Upper East Side, so he bikes through the park to school and back. Sometimes he stops at Rossleigh Court, comes up and tells Carola about the pain in his back. She has him try a few experiments. She always reminds him of the most important point: Harry, she says, these exercises will only work if you focus on your breathing.

An expert comes in to value her German furniture and china. There's the 17th century armoire, the walnut sideboard, the twelve Meissen plates from 1840. Shortly after, she lets grandson Alan, a lawyer, set up a living will. She signs the document stating that she doesn't want to be kept alive by machines. She wants to spend her final days at home, not in a hospital. She doesn't want to be artificially fed. She doesn't want artificial respiration.

There's a new drug on the streets and they call it "crack." Just breathe in once and immediately you'll feel the greatest sense of euphoria. All you need is a pipe and a lighter and some crystallized cocaine. After just ten seconds, you feel completely high. It lasts five minutes, then it's over, but your happiness will be so great that it's almost impossible not to become addicted. In reference to the phrase "to crack a whip," dealers now stand on New York street corners and move one arm in a pantomime of whipping. To make the high more intense, the pipe is short, so crack smokers often burn their mouths and people recognize their "crack lips." Crack users also show heavy breathing issues. Experts talk about "the crack lung." The US government is fighting a "War on Drugs" now, and some say it seems more like a war against those who can't let go of crack.[97]

At 251 Central Park West, a company called Orwell Management takes over the building. Some of the tenants say that nobody in the company is or ever was named Orwell. They're just using the name to emphasize how happy they will be to use all techniques of surveillance available to them. And indeed, in this new Orwellian era, management finds out that Carola's running a business in her private apartment. Because that's illegal, they threaten to evict her. They don't succeed, but for a while Carola's clients will have to whisper when they walk into the lobby. They also have to take the service elevator.

Sometimes her client Shelley stops by for a cup of tea. They're sitting in the kitchen. Shelley recommends a book to Carola: *Solitude*. Its author, psychoanalyst Anthony Storr, writes about living alone. He says that long-lasting intimate relationships are far too often seen as the only foundation for a happy existence. Storr stresses the many non-intimate relationships which are just as key to a fulfilling life. He points at relationships with neighbors, acquaintances, friends, co-workers. Intimate relationships, he notes, are "*one* center" around which a human life revolves, not "*the* center." And extraordinary people have always gone through periods of loneliness. Their lives still had purpose.[98] The breathing expert likes *Solitude* a lot.

In 1991 Carola takes a plane to France. In Paris 40 students of mindfulness gather before her to learn more about the art of breathing. She introduces them to straws. She asks them to tap themselves and to tap each other. One woman complains that the tapping felt "traumatic" to her. Another student asks Carola what she thought of that woman's remarks. She replies that she would recommend not hitting oneself. In general, people should show more patience, she says, both with themselves and others. Simply wait a little longer. It helps to think of crying babies. Once a baby stops crying, you can't put it down too abruptly. You have to wait until it really has settled. How do you know when? Pay attention to the baby's breathing.

Charlotte Selver, Charlöttchen, has also lost her husband. On the wall of her living room there are calligraphed lines by the German poet Rainer Maria Rilke. "Breath, breath, you invisible poem! / Sheer space inhaled by us, / exchanged for our small breathing. Counterbalance / in which I swing into myself, and become." Her great love Charles died on September 15, 1991. His ashes are buried on Green Gulch Farm, Muir Beach, California.[99] Charlotte is 90 years old. She also keeps teaching. Her students say that she gets younger every year. Eight years later, she's going to get married again.[100]

Carola stumbles over a rug in her apartment. She falls and breaks her hip. But she manages to crawl to the telephone to get help. She'll point out later that only her work enabled her to save herself.

Orwell seems to have given up. Carola's clients go back to using the distinguished kind of elevator. They admire Carola more than ever. Her gentleness, her friendliness. None of the exasperating conflicts people go through ever seem to happen to her.

Such conflicts also take place in the studio, though, even among these mindful breathers. There's one student, who, on a sunny day, wants the blinds to be lowered. It's important, she says. The light's distracting her. And everyone knows that this is really about the lady's ego, not about matters of light. She wants to be seen and heard. She wants to have her needs noticed. Then the blinds come down and there's this almost imperceptible smile on Carola's face that seems to say she knows what this is all about.

Then they go quiet again. They lie on their stomachs. They lift a leg. And lower the leg. And lift it again. Always the same leg. Don't forget to breathe.

Shelley's standing in front of Carola. Carola's looking at her. Shelley feels as if the work up here has given her more space inside her body. The feeling emerges when she's been quiet for a really long time, so long that it really seems too long, and has remained quiet nonetheless. That's when the space within her expands. It makes Shelley happy. She's tried all sorts of things before, Feldenkrais and Rolfing, the Alexander technique and something called antigymnastics. Only here, in the Studio of Physical Re-Education, has she found what she was looking for. And now Carola, looking at Shelley, says: "Shelley, your arms are so muscle-bound." Shelley knows this isn't meant as a compliment. She looks down. She looks to the right and to the left. Then she goes home and looks at herself in the mirror. It's true. Her arms should be hanging down in the way people's arms usually do, but they don't. These arms aren't relaxed enough. They don't hang. They're "muscle-bound." The breathing instructor sees everything.

Carola now charges 40 dollars for 90 minutes. You drop off the money in an envelope on the sideboard. A female member of the Rockefeller clan is among her clients. Next to the envelope she always leaves flowers, freshly cut, from the gardens of the family residence. Some students don't have to pay if Carola notices that they can't afford her rates.

After reading her book, people often think that everything revolves around breathing. That isn't the case. First, it's important to loosen the body. Only this will allow you to breathe freely. Even just relaxing your eyes is going to take time. It can take the entire 90 minutes. Carola's sitting on a stool, her chin resting in her hand. She's watching her clients experiment with their eyes. First you need to sense what the upper eyelids are feeling. Then the lower eyelids. Then the outer corners of your eyes. Then the inner corners. Good. Keep working. Try to see what it feels like when the eyelids are touching. Then it might be time to call it a day.

After the course she sometimes starts chatting. She tells stories about her parents, who, travelling back from Egypt, once met the King of Siam on a train. She talks about the elegant silk curtains she had in her first Berlin studio. She relates how, before the Hitler years, she was once summoned to the "Stork of Berlin," the most prominent gynecologist of his time. The Stork's wife was awfully ill. And Carola did something very simple: she made the Stork's wife lower her body into the waters of Wannsee, and right away the fever came down. Carola also tells her clients that before the war her brother Heinz had a sailboat in Marseille. One day he sailed away on it into the blue Mediterranean Sea. Sailed away, just like that, and never returned. Historical records don't support the accuracy of this story. One client looks at Carola and feels certain that some kind of light is emanating from the breathing instructor's body.

Fig. 10: Carola Speads (1995). Portrait by Robert Ullman.

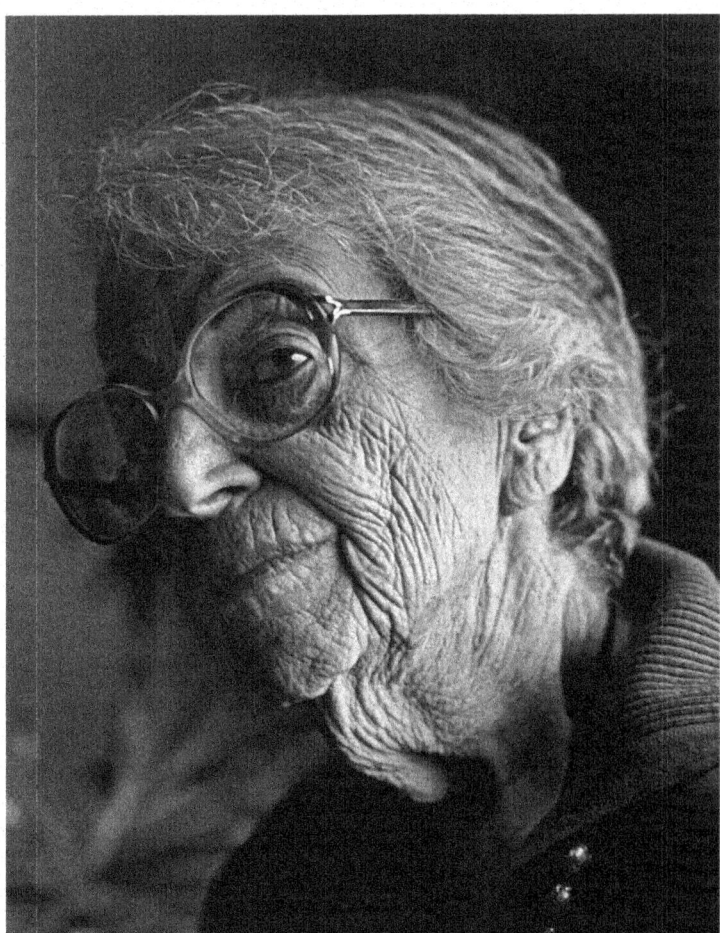

The world where you just can't breathe isn't too far from Carola's studio. You go up fifteen blocks, then you turn right toward East Harlem. At 100th Street smoke from diesel busses and garbage trucks drifts up and enters people's apartments and then their pulmonary systems. These fumes turn children into asthmatics and make their noses bleed. They transform them into weak, coughing patients. Further up, in the South Bronx, it's the same. Asthma grips entire families. Children are playing here, running around as they do everywhere. For many of them, however, any physical exertion can lead to the next asthma attack.

None of this is particularly new. What's different is that people in Harlem and the South Bronx get together to fight pollution. In 1988 they found WE ACT, an organization addressing social injustice, racism, and environmental issues as interconnected problems. It's not an accident, they say, that so many trucks and busses are passing through Harlem, many more than through other parts of the city. It's an effect of "environmental racism." In some parts of New York, there are opera houses; in others, garbage dumps and bus depots. WE ACT tells people: "Don't just breathe this all in."[101]

And this doesn't just illuminate a local problem. By the turn of the 21st century, the number of asthma patients worldwide is rising dramatically. Soon there will be 150 million, and the number of annual deaths in the hundreds of thousands. The cause of the disease is still unclear. There are fewer asthmatics in highly polluted Athens than in the clean air of New Zealand. The ratio is higher on the Maldives than in Europe. Scientists point out that there are 100,000 potentially asthma-inducing house mites on one square meter of carpeting. Others discover that the number of siblings influences the likelihood of getting asthma. The fewer siblings you have, the higher the probability you're going to turn into an asthmatic. Or is it the other way around? Conflicting studies back up both claims. Researchers prove that unhealthy eating habits trigger asthma – and before long, that hypothesis, too, is called into question. Maybe the German cockroach isn't guilty after all, it turns out, maybe stress is to blame, maybe drug addiction, maybe weight issues. Climate change leads to a rise in allergens. Experts observe that asthma, previously a disease of the upper classes, has become an affliction of the poor.[102]

Other experts question the very concept of "asthma." The patterns of the illness seem so unclear and the links to other diseases so intricate.

Studying the global ecological crisis, scientists analyze the seven million annual deaths caused by air pollution: lung cancer, strokes, and heart attacks induced by breathing in the exhaust of automobiles, factories, garbage incinerators, or wood being burned for private cooking or heating. The air quality is worst in the Middle East, in Africa, in Southeast Asia. Big cities are particularly deadly. Only in the world's most affluent places has air quality improved.[103]

Carola has been observing her body for almost a century. How warm it is and how cold, how it breathes, where it feels tight or loose. She has always taken detailed notes. And now, in 1995, she experiences a stroke that is going to change her life. One side of her body is paralyzed, and, because her chest is affected, she can only speak with great difficulty. The studio closes down. A nursing home is her new residence.

In the home, she sits in a wheelchair and refuses to take her pills. One of her students comes to visit and pushes her into the garden. She asks whether Carola is making use of her own teachings. Carola shakes her head. She's a stubborn, passive institutional patient who doesn't accept anything that could help her. Eight years ago, she coauthored an article in an academic volume on geriatric care. In the piece she explored how mindful breathing can help people master the challenges of old age. How it enables you to fight lethargy and sorrow and find a more positive outlook on life.[104] As a patient, though, she's giving up. She stops talking. It might be too hard for her. Or maybe she's simply ashamed.

Carola, her students feel, must return to 251 Central Park West. She simply must teach again, and Carola's daughter must help. But she can't. Dorothea Fraade, 72 by now, has always been the most dutiful daughter, but she has a husband who's a stroke patient as well and needs her permanent care. Still her mother's clients don't give in. Isn't there anything she could do? Dorothea declines. But the studio must open up again. There is simply no other way and so Carola eventually returns to the tenth floor of Rossleigh Court. Paid for by the studio clients, a nurse called Dolly moves in with her. Carola's classes resume.

There's one more thing, the clients feel, that needs to be resolved: the conflict with Charlotte Selver. They know how difficult this will be. But they also feel that these two women simply have to make up. And so one of Carola's clients, Mary Alice Roche, takes on the mission. She first studied mindfulness with Charlotte and then turned to Carola and found her breath. Mary Alice talks to Charlotte. A woman as opinionated as she is harmony-loving, Charlotte agrees to attend. So does Carola – though it's hard to read her facial expressions these days.

Half a century after their dramatic separation, the two gymnastics teachers meet again. One mindfulness student pushes Charlotte, in her wheelchair, from the elevator into the studio and stops in front of Carola's wheelchair. Carola gets flowers. Charlotte talks. Carola doesn't. It's unclear whether she would if she could. Looking back later, one witness will remember that Carola showed absolutely no sign of friendliness or forgiveness. Another Carola student swears that it was a very warm and friendly reunion, a true reconciliation after all those years. The student, however, wasn't present that day.

The classes continue. There's Carola Speads, paralyzed and mute. And there are her clients, all dressed in white, sitting on the ground in front of her. Carola's giving signals with her left hand. This is the hand she can still move. She taps her finger against her temple to show them that they need to concentrate. If they misunderstand her, she hits the little table on her wheelchair with her hand. She gives them the thumbs-up signal when they look relaxed and open. When they seem tense, Carola's face cramps into a grimace. When a student's hand seems too loose, she demonstrates with her own hand that a hand is a living thing and not just a flabby appendage dangling from the body. She touches her knee to show her students that this would be a good time to lift a knee. When she feels that they're all in good shape and that the time has come to sit and breathe, she moves her lips forward, just a little bit, and her clients read the signal. Silence. Patience. They sit. They breathe. And Carola's breathing with them.

6. Speads Work

It's early in the Trump Era. You have no idea that a pandemic is about to affect the breathing of millions, if not billions, on the planet. You do know that an asthmatic African American New Yorker named Eric Garner recently died in a chokehold. A white New York City police officer didn't let go, though Garner repeatedly said: "I can't breathe." A movement named Black Lives Matter will soon raise new questions about bodily experience, racism, and everyday life.[105]

You're visiting from Germany, and you're sitting with Steven Fraade and Jonathan Fraade in a large living room of a suburban house in Connecticut. These are two of Carola Spitz's three grandsons. They are serene men in their sixties. On June 26, 1999, their grandmother died after a second, more intense stroke. She was still teaching just two months before her death. Now she lives on as the subject of the conversation: as grandmother, teacher, German Jewish refugee. You're looking through the picture window and you spot deer moving through the woods. Every workday Jonathan Fraade leaves this house, drives to the Westport train station, gets on a Metro North train, and gets off about an hour later at Grand Central to go to work in Manhattan, as Senior Client Portfolio Manager in the Global Fixed Income, Currency & Commodities Group at J.P. Morgan. Today he has taken a day off. His brother Steven drove down this morning from New Haven. He's the Mark Taper Professor of the History of Judaism at Yale.

During your conversation, the three of you explore what kind of grandmother Carola Spitz was. You end up discussing "Königsberger Klopse," the German dish featuring meatballs and capers in white sauce.

She made these occasionally. Steven and Jonathan are trying to figure out whether that held any significance for the kind of grandmother she was. It turns out that she strove to keep her work and private life separate. And the grandsons agree that her Studio of Physical Re-Education was far more important to her than "Königsberger Klopse" could ever have been. They say that Otto, their grandfather, may have had the warmer personality of the two. He appeared at school events and music recitals. Carola taught in her studio. Maybe she wanted to and maybe she had to. Jonathan talks about the bitter poverty that many German Jewish refugees found themselves in, in their old age, in New York City. It was different for their grandparents.

Boxes are sitting on a table in this living room. They contain letters and diaries of Carola Joseph/Spitz/Speads, bills, scrapbooks, notes of breathing lessons. There's not much information about the clients. The grandsons have thrown out a lot of documents referring to them. They had assumed that nobody would ever be interested. You do disagree with that assumption. Oh yes, you do. In the boxes you find, among other things, documents about blood donations made by the Spitzs in the late 1940s, the May 1970 edition of *Mademoiselle*, and a photo album documenting a Black Forest hiking trip in the early 1920s.

After your meeting with the grandsons, you spend the night at the Bridgeport Holiday Inn. The Yale Center for Sleep Medicine keeps some rooms in this hotel. Extreme snorers sleep here. Polysomnographic technicians monitor their complex breathing.[106] It seems, however, as if these patients aren't snoring in the rooms right next to yours. Therefore you're fully rested when you take the Metro North to Grand Central in the morning. You expect that Carola's life will reveal itself to you in New York City.

Walk around in Washington Heights. Climb steep hills. Look at the Hudson, the George Washington Bridge, New Jersey. Turn around and go back to Fort Washington Avenue. On this Saturday almost every male passerby is wearing a kippah. In the school yard of Public School No. 187, though, mostly bare-headed kids hang around the basketball court. On the other side of the street, there's 660 Ft. Washington, Carola, Otto, and Dorothea's first residence in New York City. The moment you stop in front of it, a generously tattooed young woman emerges from the building. Her hair gleams pink.

Walk down the hill toward the subway. You'll notice the line that Broadway still seems to be drawing between the Jewish, upper-middle-class Heights, and the formerly Irish, now Latino, not so upper-, though still middle-class Heights. On this side of Broadway, you stop in front of Mount Sinai Synagogue and read the sign referring to Ezra Schwartz, Senior Rabbi, and Mordecai Schnaidman, Rabbi Emeritus, and on the other side of Broadway there's La Cabaña Salvadoreña offering "comidas tipicas" and right next door from La Cabaña you see Dr. R. De La Cruz's acupuncture clinic. Climb the hill to St. Nicholas Avenue. Take the subway at 191st Street, just like Carola used to, in the 1940s. Get out at 81st Street and turn from Central Park West into the park. You're just minutes south of the body of water which one of Carola's 1950s letters to Elsa Gindler described in so much detail. It is now called Jacqueline Kennedy Onassis Reservoir. Find your way to Belvedere Castle. Walk around Turtle Pond. You're looking for a tree that Carola's clients planted for her. You're looking for a plaque, a sign. You don't find it. You walk around Turtle Pond once more and you'll later learn that there is indeed a tree for her, a black birch, producing oxygen for breathing New Yorkers, but no sign bearing her name.

You don't just want to look for traces of the past in New York. You're also curious about the present. There's a breathing teacher here you very much wanted to meet: Belisa Vranich, known as Dr. Belisa. She says that her breathing techniques will take you towards mental and physical health. One of her specialties is "Rock'n'Roll Breath." Dr. Belisa warns you not to breathe incorrectly. Vertically, for instance. You tried in vain to make an appointment with Dr. Belisa. Her teachings promise a larger hippocampus, a more vital temporoparietal junction, and a strengthened brainstem.

Fig. 11: 251 Central Park West.

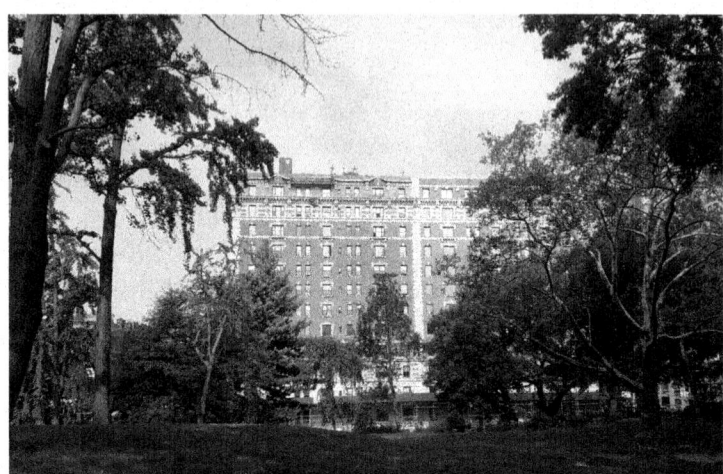

Dan Brulé, a former soldier, also plays a role in this business. He recommends hypopressive breathing to intensify circulation, flatten the stomach, and cure incontinence, constipation, and sexual problems. As a hypopressive breather, you breathe in, you breathe out, and then you pretend to breathe in again, but you don't, thus expanding your chest, holding it for ten seconds, and then you breathe in.[107]

Breathe like Dan Brulé. Breathe like Dr. Belisa. Or walk a few blocks and have coffee with Carola Spitz's niece Frances and her husband Harry, on West End Avenue. Take out your note pad and record that Fritz Spitz, Otto's brother, at some point left all the work in his clothing store to his wife Adele and that Adele was able to count on Hercules, a long-term staff member (Hercules had Greek roots). Put away your notepad. Take a walk on the Upper West Side with Frances and a large pug whose panting doesn't sound healthy at all. The dog is visiting, just like you. Usually, he lives on the Upper East Side with one of Frances' and Harry's sons. You cross the first street next to Frances' building and the pug refuses to take another step. A case of vertical breathing? Maybe.

Say good-bye to Frances and the pug and walk back to 251 Central Park West. Take the elevator to the twelfth floor, two floors above the former Studio of Physical Re-Education. Here you meet another dog. To calm this nervous pet down and establish a personal relationship, Broadway actress Joanna Glushak tells you to hand the dog a piece of chicken. And you do. Joanna has offered to show you her apartment and the view. She has so many stories to tell about life in Rossleigh Court. Unfortunately, she's very clear that most of these stories could never ever be told in your – or anyone's – book. Currently Joanna's in the cast of *Warpaint*, a play about the rivalry between make-up moguls Elizabeth Arden and Helena Rubinstein. Look out of the window to enjoy the same view Carola enjoyed. It's a very cloudy day, but that doesn't matter.

On another day you meet Alan, Carola's third grandson, in his office on Madison Avenue. Just steps away, on 39th Street, are the offices of the Carl Gustav Jung Foundation. Jung wrote that the Kenyan people called the Elgonyi didn't have a single religious ritual. At daybreak, however, the Elgonyi breathed and spit on their hands, raised their hands and held them toward the sky, into the rising sun, to offer their spirit – breath – and their life force – spit – to the sun.[108] Alan Fraade is a very friendly man, but today is a busy day. At night the Elgonyi, Jung writes, do the same thing to welcome the moon. Breath and spit. Keep in mind that Jung may not have known everything about Elgonyi culture. In the evening, have dinner at Go Go Dim Sum, Chinatown, with Susan Gregory, formerly Susan Elrauch, an opera singer and long-term client of Carola's. In the morning, return to the Upper West Side. Discuss typical New York real estate questions about rent-controlled leases, rent-stabilized leases, and market rent. Realize that, today, the dancers, therapists, and singers who used to breathe at Carola's place would never be able to afford an apartment on the Upper West Side. Realize also that all these points aren't getting you any closer to the heart of Carola's world. That heart consisted of "the work." Gindler work. That was her life.

Get on a plane, then, live your life, and then stretch out on a mat on the floor of a villa in the Berlin suburb of Grunewald. Don't look out of the window. There are trees, and their branches are moving in the wind, but the course instructor tells you not to "travel." On your ribcage there's a sack the size of a tennis ball. Underneath this sack are your lungs. There are about a dozen other people in the room with you, also on mats. There is a sack on everyone. It's an experiment. The instructor speaks softly. But she knows what she wants. Someone, not you, thank God, put the sack on their belly, not the ribcage. That must be corrected. Everyone needs to have the sack in the same position. There was no sack there before, says the instructor. Now there is. What has changed? How does that feel? Nobody answers. Everyone's alone with their sack.

You signed up for this course months ago. It's a seven-day event: "Introduction to Gindler Work." The course fee was 350 Euros. This is the first day. You have to do this. You want to understand Carola, the Gindler student. Nobody teaches "Speads Work" today. Carola did not begin her own tradition. It had to be Gindler work. The course is taught in the headquarters of the Jacoby Gindler Foundation. The Foundation has the explicit purpose of keeping alive the work of Heinrich Jacoby, a Lebensreform music teacher, and Elsa Gindler. You've heard from a member of the Berlin bodywork community that the Foundation might focus too much on Jacoby and doesn't seem all that loyal to Gindler's teachings. You still signed up. This must be the closest thing to working with Carola.

Now the instructor tells you to move the sack from your ribcage to the ground. The sack was there. Now it's gone. How does that feel, the instructor asks. What has changed?

Remind yourself not to look out the window. After an excruciatingly long time the instructor tells you to move the sack back onto your body. Don't put it in the same spot, though. Move it one sackbreadth further up in the direction of your clavicle. There was no sack there before. Now there's a sack there. How does that feel? Don't lose focus. You're in the right place. You really need to learn more about breathing. If a sack's necessary, then there really has to be a sack. Don't think about all the other stuff. Issues with the kids. No. Being a better father. It's probably too late anyway. Why is it always too late for everything? Don't look at the grey sky. The branches in the wind. Or would you call those twigs? Don't think about the difference between branches and twigs.

Now, because of branches, twigs, the sky, kids, and fatherhood, you have missed putting the sack back on the ground. You just barely heard the instructor announce what she wanted you to do, so you reached for the sack abruptly and of course you know that this kind of quick, unfocused movement Gindler people don't approve of. The instructor is uncomfortably close. The sack was there. Now it's not. How does that feel?

Earlier today the instructor caught you napping. You know that in Manhattan, in Carola's studio, dozing off was perfectly fine. Gindler hadn't minded either. Here, in the Jacoby Gindler Foundation Headquarters, there's a no sleeping rule. Better to keep your eyes open, the instructor said. She has her eye on you and you know it. Maybe she doesn't like the way you dressed for class. One of the guidelines supplied by the instructor asked students to turn up in white leggings. Yesterday you dashed out, minutes before the stores closed, and bought a pair of grey jogging pants, at Uniqlo.

Some of the questions are interesting, though. When you were lying on the studio floor this morning, the instructor asked: What does the floor do? And you thought about that for quite some time. Then she asked whether there was something between the arms. And whether the head was connected to the neck. These questions really shed light on things you've always taken for granted. Maybe Carola asked these kinds of questions too. They didn't sound spiritual or poetic, just exploratory, scientific.

The sack and its sackness. You imagined a different kind of course. In your mind you had this Netflix image of Carola's studio, of eloquent opera singers and cosmopolitan art historians and Rockefeller heiresses bringing freshly cut flowers. You imagined their silences, their conversations, their tears, their laughter, and you pictured this scene when they left the studio, feeling kind of high, coming out of the elevator, surely not the service one, with these elastic movements, waving to the doorman and then, maybe, taking a sprightly walk around the Jacqueline Kennedy Onassis Reservoir. In contrast, this course here seems frightfully German.

But now, finally, the sack has reached your clavicle. And the instructor calls it a day. Day one of seven. But she tells you not to get up right away. She asks each member of the group to loll a bit, against the wall. Like a lolling cat. Lolling, though, seems utterly impossible to you. No, you will not loll. You get up. Just like that. Not catlike at all. To save face in the Gindler community, you act as if you'd return tomorrow. You put on your shoes, say goodbye, tell the instructor and your fellow clients that of course, as the instructor has just announced, you will show up half an hour before the course begins, because everyone will need the time to really adapt to the experience. Certainly. Walk away, fast, but not too fast, from the Jacoby Gindler Foundation premises and tell your instructor the next morning, per email, and you might want to use your phone to leave an additional message on the Foundation's answering machine, that you will not be showing up for the next six days. Hide away at home, in complete isolation.

Or think again. It's really not all that original to mock mindful bodywork, particularly if you're speaking from a privileged white male perspective. When women developed these techniques, around the beginning of the 20th century, they did so to subvert male-dominated practices of the body: medical science, for instance, which defined the male body as the norm and treated female bodily experiences as abnormal. In breathing together, in sensing together, women introduced new forms of intellectual exchange. Women gymnastics instructors were insulted as "ethereal she-goats" in the early 20th century, by men.[109] Marxist philosopher Ernst Bloch made fun of them, calling them "bourgeois and weird," and said they had no idea of hunger, dust, and smoke, no concept of the "squalor" plaguing the working class.[110]

Like Bloch, you didn't get it. If you'd really wanted to follow Gindler/Speads, you should have known that it was your own breath that was teaching the course, not an instructor you had issues with. You had expected knowledge to be passed to you from above, and you didn't realize that the Gindler method of self-exploration works as a network instead.[111] And Gindler, as we know, was more than familiar with the "squalor" foregrounded by Ernst Bloch. In fact, she discovered mindfulness precisely because she was from the working class and excluded from the privileged career paths of her time.

In the Berlin years, one Berta Bobath was one of Carola's first students – and she later became a globally known pioneer of physiotherapy. Bobath applied Carola's methods to her own work with children and young adults with cerebral palsy. In her bodywork she approached these clients as though she were dancing with them: slowly, in a careful, exploratory mode, not following her own, Berta Bobath's, rhythm, only the rhythm the clients themselves suggested. It was Carola Speads, Bobath wrote, who had taught her how to handle coordination and breathing.[112]

If such ideas don't seem like revolutionary concepts, maybe your concept of what's revolutionary needs to change. The techniques developed by Gindler, Speads, and Bobath created a new intellectual subculture, dominated by women, which spread from Berlin to the United States, Israel, France, the United Kingdom, into physiotherapy, psychoanalysis, gestalt therapy. This nameless work had emancipatory power for women, for the sick, the disabled, the traumatized – a kind of power, though, that Marxist theorists don't usually see.[113]

And then there's Mike Korzinski, son of a Volvo dealer and a psychotherapist from New Jersey. He tells you, from London, in a video call, about his memories of Sunday mornings spent with Carola Speads and of his own therapeutic work with victims of torture. He talks about this one man who had been mauled both by the men of the Shah and the men of Ayatollah Khomeini, and whose body was so foreign to him that he kept his arms wrapped tightly around his chest. This man was afraid of breathing, Mike Korzinski says. To work with him, first on breathing and then on perceiving the body as a safe space again: that was a step in coming through trauma. Mike also talks about his father and his memories of war, about the ashes in Hiroshima and Nagasaki, and about the studio on Central Park West. Then he gets up. He puts a gymnastics ball on his head and moves around the room. You can tell that he used to be a ballet dancer. He laughs while walking around, just like they laughed at 251 Central Park West when something had gone wrong, or an embarrassing bodily sound had been emitted in the stillness of the studio. Mike sits back down at his desk, next to which he keeps his guitars, and talks about the newest discoveries in the field of trauma therapy. He mentions limbic research. He says that Carola was ahead of her time. She was doing all these things back then already, Mike says: therapeutic work that bypassed the frontal cortex. And yet nobody knows her now, Mike says, because she was so principled and never combined her work with anything else. And Mike says that he knows why that was the case. She was always certain, he points out, that it was only breathing, mindful breathing, that had helped her get her husband out of the Berlin prison. The work had saved Otto's life and Dorothea's life and her own life. And because of that, changing "the work" would have seemed like betrayal to her.

Mike Korzinski's enthusiasm is catching. Some moments, Carola Joseph/Spitz/Speads seems like a forgotten 20th century heroine to you. She was one of those modern migrants who managed, in spite of all obstacles and tragedies, to find a niche in a new culture, a new economy, and transformed her own knowledge and skills. In contrast to Charlotte Selver, she didn't make it to the renowned New School for Social Research. But she did run her own independent research institute: the Studio for Physical Re-Education. Instead of poeticizing or romanticizing her method, she cultivated its quietness and its depth almost until the new millennium – and she did so in a monstrously capitalist city where there's almost no room for quietness and depth.

On closer inspection, though, this picture of a subversive immigrant intellectual doesn't seem all that convincing. Doubtlessly Carola Spitz lived through a time of enormous uncertainty. Nonetheless she belonged to the economic elite of German Jewish refugees. One of the witnesses interviewed for this book called her a "princess" and said she was "to the manor born." Two interviewees stated that Carola perhaps had too much of the sophisticated lady to her. They talked about how disappointed she was that her adopted daughter had married a man who didn't meet her, Carola's, social expectations. (He was also from Washington Heights, but from the wrong side of Broadway.) And even in the 1950s, learning to breathe with a view of Central Park was something only the affluent could afford. In today's context, her studio seems like the perfect, alarming symbol of the hypergentrified metropolis: an oasis of luxury, far removed from its urban environment.

In addition Carola strikes us as a completely apolitical figure. Hannah Arendt, who also lived on the Upper West Side, turned her anger about the Holocaust into political philosophy. And if the comparison to this singular thinker seems unfair, we could turn our attention to another refugee in Carola's neighborhood, just a few blocks from her, on Central Park West: Hertha Nathorff, a former Berlin physician. Nathorff never managed to get the papers to practice in New York, but she compensated for this by working for numerous social justice projects.[114] Finally, edgy Charlotte Selver, poetic and idiosyncratic, who passed away in 2003 at the age of 102, seems to have had much more rebellious power than Carola Speads. And even mindfulness itself, a subversive and feminist practice in Elsa Gindler's studio, we can't really appreciate anymore. Rather, we see it as an element of neoliberalism – or, as one expert has it, as "the new capitalist spirituality." Today's mindful individuals, scholars explain, are really just managing the stress of an ever more unjust economic system. Instead of addressing the system's failures, mindfulness talk cajoles us into self-improvement programs.[115] If you follow these lines of thinking, exporting German bodywork to Manhattan can't really be seen as a liberatory act.

It's very much a matter of context, then, whether we categorize this protagonist as a heroic figure. She didn't change the world. But the world also gave her little opportunity to do so. We might want to take our cue from Gindler and Speads, stop looking for rebellious grandeur, and simply notice what was. This breathing expert's life invites us to pay attention to things we usually take for granted. Her story sheds light on the 20th century, which destroyed and limited so many lives and made so many biographies seem downright absurd.

Carola's private and public history illuminates both enormous privilege and complete disenfranchisement. It contains elegant Berlin bourgeois lifestyles and aggressive German antisemitism; it connects luxurious self-examination and industrialized mass murder. It's a history of silencing. It shows how people distance themselves from the world or take an almost grotesquely microscopic view of reality, simply because it's the only way to keep living a meaningful life.

And Carola's story takes us to this: that in the summer of 1942, in Amsterdam, her mother, Paula Joseph, probably heard the rumors that Jews deported to Poland were killed there. People listening to the BBC learned this. On June 29, 1942 a Dutch homemaker named Aaltje de Vries-Bouwes wrote in her diary that, in Eastern Europe, since May 1940, 700,000 Jews had been murdered "with machine guns or in a gas chamber." De Vries-Bouwes said she'd heard that these people had to dig their own graves before these mass executions, and that up to 90 people were killed at the same time in the gas chambers.[116] On September 26, 1942 Paula Joseph sent a Red Cross message to her daughter Carola in New York. She stated that she was "ready for everything that seemed inevitable."

On December 30, 1942, Paula Joseph was deported from Amsterdam to Westerbork, a camp close to the Dutch-German border. Paula Joseph arrived there during a brief lull in deportations. Two weeks before she arrived the last transport had departed, on December 12. Deportations resumed on January 11. On that day Paula Joseph and 749 others were forced on a train to Auschwitz.[117]

In Manhattan, on July 8, 1945, Carola Spitz received a telegram from Amsterdam, sent by one Joseph Meyer. He informed her about Paula Joseph's deportation from Westerbork in December 1942 and her deportation from there, "destination unknown," in January 1943. On September 29, 1951, the Dutch Red Cross wrote to New York, confirming these dates and specifying Auschwitz as the terminal point of this transport. This letter said that Paula Joseph "must be assumed to have been asphyxiated there on 14th January 1943." Carola also learned that her brother had been deported from the French camp Drancy to Auschwitz, on August 31, 1942, and that he had also lost his life there.

Very few people in her circle seem to have known these details. Very briefly Carola Spitz wrote to Elsa Gindler about what she knew right after the war. Apart from this correspondence, there is no evidence that Carola Spitz had any conversations with other people about these events.

We can only speculate as to how the fate of her mother and her brother affected her. A comparison might help. Margaret Mahler, four years Carola's senior, a psychoanalyst from Vienna and, like her, a refugee in New York, had also tried to save her mother's life by writing letters from the United States to Europe. She was also unsuccessful. After the war Mahler had also waited a painfully long time to hear about what happened and had then learned that her mother had been killed in Auschwitz. Much later she described the nightmarish experience of unsuccessfully trying to save her mother's life and the severe depression which the news of her death had triggered in her. We can assume that Margret Mahler was a professional when it came to having conversations. She was a psychoanalyst, after all. Late in her life, though, she reported that decades had passed and she had only told one single person in New York about her mother's fate.[118]

Carola Spitz may have found herself in a similar situation. Being interviewed by her grandson Alan when she was 88, she said tersely that her mother had "perished" and that her mother's cousin Erna, also a refugee in the Netherlands, had survived. Then she changed the subject. The only documents in her papers reflecting the loss she had experienced are the letters she and Otto exchanged with West German reparation authorities and lawyers. Her attorney Walter Schwarz had informed Carola Spitz that she could claim reparations for her mother's deportation and death.[119] She had followed up on this. Responding to her claim, West Berlin authorities decided in 1959 to compensate her for Paula Joseph's suffering in the Netherlands and in Auschwitz with the amount of 1200 German marks. At that time a new VW Beetle cost four times as much.[120]

In this breathing expert's life story, we need to consider that in matters of breathing, German doctors, businessmen, and military personnel had cooperated since the summer of 1939. They had planned and debated and finally decided to murder human beings by poisoning them through their respiratory systems. Initially these German experts had planned the killing of the incurably ill and the disabled. The first gas chamber murders of patients took place in an SS camp in Poznan in November

1939. They were suffocated with carbon monoxide. From then on, teams of German scientists, SS men, and administration staff collaborated in a town called Brandenburg to plan additional killings of disabled adults and children in gas chambers. After the 1942 Wannsee Conference, the mass murder of Jews with the substance Zyklon B began in the gas chambers of Auschwitz and other camps. The usage of combustion engines in the extermination system is less foregrounded in historical debates. From these machines, toxic exhaust was conducted to gas chambers or the insides of trucks. These killing methods, too, emerged from decision-making processes in which German experts explored human breathing and the efficiency and availability of substances causing asphyxiation. Approximately two million victims of German violence were killed because they breathed in engine exhausts in closed rooms. Around one million people suffocated because their bodies took in Zyklon B. About 100,000 were murdered with carbon monoxide.[121]

It seems inappropriate to explore such matters in a book that also contains such whimsical anecdotes as the story of Hans Surén, with his loincloth, his oiled body, and his oddball ideas about self-massage. But it would also appear inaccurate to tell the story of Carola Spitz and her family and fail to place it in its historical context. A history of German discourses on the body, like the one sketched in the preceding pages, must reflect the continuity between ideas popular in early 20th century Germany and the system of extermination devised from the 1930s onwards. There are inextricable links between German gymnasts, always attentive to the rhythm of the breath, and meticulously planned mass murders by asphyxiation. The Holocaust is rooted in a contrast German culture created: between the strong "Aryan" body and the weak body of the "Other," the latter to be attacked and weakened even further without ever showing mercy. These links cannot be ignored. Carola Spitz's life brings them to light.

And, finally, there's Dorothea, Carola's and Otto's daughter, a woman who never spent more than ten minutes on the phone. She was down-to-earth, thrifty, always on time. Every morning at 9:30 a.m. she called her mother. They talked in German. After high school Dorothea had attended Hunter College, then worked as a nutritionist in the New York City school system. Then she married a Jewish New Yorker, Bert Fraade, and became a homemaker. They had a modest little cabin in Sherman, Connecticut. In that cabin she sometimes turned on the vacuum cleaner at six in the morning. Every day she put on a bathing cap and went for a swim in Candlewood Lake. When she was in Manhattan, it went without saying that she took the bus, not a taxi. Until the end of her life, she had a pretty strong German accent. Whenever anyone asked her about it, she always replied: "Accent? What accent?"

Dorothea Fraade noticed that Jewishness was important to her sons. All three of them, Steven, Jonathan, and Alan, married Jewish women and sent their children, her grandchildren, to Jewish schools. She had been raised in a Jewish family that had pork on the dinner table and Christmas trees as a given. Her aunt Adele, Fritz Spitz's wife, had stopped smoking every year for the duration of Yom Kippur, and started again the day after. This was as intense as religiosity got in that generation. Her sons' religious beliefs surprised her. She saw their practicing of Jewishness as a phase that would certainly pass.

She was wrong. But she didn't question her children's decisions. And then she herself began to live a more explicitly Jewish life. When Johnny, her youngest, had turned eleven, she took on a fulltime job. She worked as a secretary in a Washington Heights synagogue, and those who knew her remember how she fought for women's equality in the temple. She stayed in the job until she was 81 years old. And she kept working. She volunteered for the Young Men's and Women's Hebrew Organization on Nagle Avenue in Washington Heights.

Dorothea Fraade organized family reunions for the holidays, the Jewish ones, like Passover, and the secular ones, like Thanksgiving or the Fourth of July. She always invited her mother and father, her uncle and aunt, her sons and their partners, as well as Frances, her rebellious cousin, and Frances's cousin Harry, their kids, their grandchildren. It was always important to her that everyone showed up.

For the party celebrating her 85th birthday, Dorothea, once known as Thea, and then, for the longest time, as "Dotty," was planning to give a speech. She had just recovered from an illness and had noted down her remarks on a yellow pad. She wore a flowery blouse and a beige jacket and carried a cane in her hand as she stepped out of the Fort Washington Avenue building into which she had moved with Carola and Otto 68 years before.

It was June 15, 2008. The party took place on the Upper East Side, at Compass Restaurant on 70th Street, where Broadway crosses Amsterdam Avenue. On that day a presidential candidate named Barack Obama gave a speech in Chicago in which he advised Americans to spend more time with their kids. Dorothea Fraade, born a subject of Reichspräsident Friedrich Ebert, spent time with her children and grandchildren that night, and with a few friends, and she used her own speech to address how grateful she was to all the people around her. She mentioned that somebody had said how unlucky she had been to have three sons and no daughter. And she said how that was so wrong. She said her sons were wonderful and so were her daughters-in-law and her grandchildren. She concluded her speech by thanking her family and friends for coming – and thanking her sons for not postponing the party even though she'd asked them to, several times, in fact. She said she was happy they hadn't listened to her. There was applause. And then the daughter of Carola Speads breathed in. There is a pause between breathing in and breathing out. During that pause, Dorothea Fraade from Washington Heights took a good look at the burning candles on her birthday cake.

Sources

This is the nonfictional account of a life and its context. As all biographies will, this one, too, promises coherence and authenticity. And yet, every account of one individual's story will emerge as incomplete and subjective and any sense of unity just some construct cobbled together by the author.[122] Add to this the mistakes every writer makes, this one certainly included, and the term "nonfiction" will appear as an awfully weak concept. I can state, however, that nowhere in this book have I fictionalized anything consciously and willingly. Every detail stems from sources and/or interviews.

The papers of Carola and Otto Spitz were central to my research. I would like to thank Steven, Alan, and Jonathan Fraade for being so generous with these resources. The following documents were particularly important: Carola Spitz's extensive, precise diaries illuminated her childhood and youth. Her work as a gymnastics instructor in the 1920s and 1930s was detailed in personal letters, in course reports about her own work and her work with Elsa Gindler, as well as in other, more unsystematic notes. In Alan Fraade's wide-ranging video interview, Carola Spitz speaks about her husband's imprisonment and her efforts to have him freed. Her papers also document the story of the family's escape, first from Germany, then from France. Paula Joseph's experiences in Amsterdam are described in her letters to New York. In these letters Carola Spitz's mother also comments on her daughter's letters from Manhattan to Amsterdam, and thus makes it possible to tell the story of the early New York years of the Spitz family. Extensive personal letters to Elsa Gindler document Carola's experiences in the 1950s, from her own private troubles to her view of Central Park and her reflections on working with clients. Postwar correspondence between German authorities and the Spitz family helped to shed light on biographical details in the postwar period and in the years of persecution and escape.

In order to explore the second half of Carola Speads' life, I used the anthology "A Glimpse of Paradise," an unpublished work produced by her students. I also interviewed experts and witnesses and I would like to thank these individuals for taking the time and for being such conscientious interviewees. Had it not been for Steven Fraade's openness and patience, this book would never have seen the light of day. For years, he made himself available for in-person conversations, Skype interviews, and dozens of e-mails. He helped in a twin capacity: as a loving chronicler of his family history and as a renowned expert on Jewish history and culture. Alan Fraade searched for and found a matchbook from Compass Restaurant; Jonathan Fraade remembered that at his mother's 85th anniversary party, a birthday cake had sat on the table and the candles had burned. But Alan and Jonathan both had so much more to report.

I could not have told the story of the Studio of Physical Re-Education without Susan Gregory's incredible support. In personal conversations, video interviews, and e-mail exchanges, she helped me wrap my mind around "the work." It was a great privilege and an enormous pleasure to interview such an undogmatic and eloquent witness and expert. Susan Gregory contributed to this account in multiple roles: as the former Susan Elrauch, as a client of Carola Speads, as a New Yorker, an opera singer, a singing teacher, and a gestalt therapist. Guided by Susan's expertise, I was able to reconstruct one of Carola's lessons in the opening chapter of this book.

I also conducted extensive interviews with bodywork expert Shelley Hainer, who in the spring of 2018 organized a reunion of Carola's former students in New York City. Phyllis Joyner contributed much to this inspiring afternoon. Frances and Harry Lester were generous hosts on West End Avenue and lively, challenging interviewees about the Spitz family history. In a long video conversation, Mike Korzinski outlined the meaning of Carola Speads' work for his family and his own therapeutic practice. Anthony Mariano, Orwell Management, New York City, generously provided the opportunity to explore 251 Central Park West from the inside. Even more generously, Joanna Glushak took the time to talk on the twelfth floor and let me look out the window. Stefan Laeng-Gilliatt agreed to an extensive conversation and kindly shared his in-depth research on Charlotte Selver. I'd also like to thank the Department of Special Research Collections, University of California, Santa Barbara, for providing access to the Charlotte Selver collection, and Robert Ullmann for opening his photo archives. Special thanks to Brad Prager (University of Missouri) for perspicacious advice and to Jim van der Laan (Illinois State University) for last-minute help. Finally, Steven Fraade's children (Shoshana Cohen-Fraade, Liora Cohen-Fraade, and Nathaniel Cohen-Fraade) helped me see the contemporary aspects of this story. In our e-mail exchanges, they expressed how much their grandmother's and their great-grandparents' stories of persecution had shaped their own identities, both personally and professionally. The vacuum cleaner droning in Sherman, Connecticut, emerged from their memories. It was more important to them, however, to call attention to their family's escape from Europe despite the bureaucratic obstacles and political barriers in the way, and to point out the parallels to the experiences of today's migrants, in the United States and at its borders.

On the other side of the Atlantic, Birgit Rohloff at the Jacoby Gindler Archive answered many questions and moved my research along. I'd also like to thank a Gindler course instructor, unnamed here, who objected to naps in the studio. Maybe she had a point. I'm grateful to Christian Heilbronn (Suhrkamp) for turning the German-language version of Carola Speads' story into *Die Atemlehrerin*. Anja Schneider, a breathing teacher in Berlin, took time for a conversation, Gabriele Franzen commented on today's Gindler work, Aurelia Ehrensperger let me read her dissertation, Sandra Fries supplied her diploma thesis. Matthias Scharer shared important work on Ruth Cohn, Katja Rother provided her scholarship on Elsa Gindler. Florence Moehl helped me understand Flora Türkel, Heidi Schönberger responded to inquiries about Carola Speads' postwar ties to Germany. Christoph Kreutzmüller and Dieter Gosewinkel explained historical background. Nurit Wenger-Varga answered questions about Dorothea Fraade's time in Switzerland. Thanks are due to Stela Dujakovic, Alexander Dunst, Richard Grasshoff, Alexandra Hartmann, Michael Heimann, Miriam Jassmeier, Frank Kelleter, Petra Meyenbrock, Wilbert Olinde, Denise Parkinson, Marie Smith, Änne Söll. Many thanks to Carolin Willeke for her research assistance and her meticulous transcriptions of Paula Joseph's letters. In conclusion let me thank Jamie Lee Searle for her fantastic editorial work.

Illustrations

Fig. 1: Carola Spitz in 1946. Photograph, United States Certificate of Naturalization. From the Papers of Carola and Otto Spitz.
Fig. 2: Client in the Studio of Physical Re-Education. Photograph by Carola Speads in unpublished Festschrift "A Glimpse of Paradise."
Fig. 3: In the Black Forest. From the Papers of Carola and Otto Spitz.
Fig. 4: Anna Hermann's students. Photograph taken for Scherl Verlag in 1926. From the Papers of Carola and Otto Spitz.
Fig. 5: Client in the Studio of Physical Re-Education. Photograph by Carola Speads in "A Glimpse of Paradise."
Fig. 6: Client in the Studio of Physical Re-Education. Photograph by Carola Speads in "A Glimpse of Paradise."
Fig. 7: Photograph of Berlin cigarette factory run by Otto Spitz. From the Papers of Carola and Otto Spitz.
Fig. 8: *Breathing: The ABC's*. Book cover. Harper & Row.
Fig. 9: Carola Speads in the studio. From "A Glimpse of Paradise."
Fig. 10: Carola Speads in 1995. Photograph by Robert Ullmann.
Fig. 11: 251 Central Park West. Photograph by the author.

Notes

The Studio of Physical Re-Education

1. These endnotes refer to published material. For unpublished documents see the chapter "Sources." In the main text of this book, quotations marks are only used when the quotation was found in a written document. Regarding "Little Germany," see: Richard Panchyk, *German New York City* (Charleston: Arcadia, 2008), 94–97.
2. For Walter Schwarz's biography: Arnold Lehmann-Richter, *Auf der Suche nach den Grenzen der Wiedergutmachung: Die Rechtsprechung zur Entschädigung für Opfer der nationalsozialistischen Verfolgung* (Berlin: BWV, 2007), 55.
3. Eric A. Goldstein and Mark A. Izeman, "Pollution," *Encyclopedia of New York City*, ed. Kenneth T. Jackson (New Haven: Yale University Press, 1995), 914–916.
4. Alberta Szalita and Darel Benaim, *The Force of Destiny* (New York: Jay Street, 2005), 105.
5. Robert A.M. Stern, Thomas Mellins, and David Fishman, *New York 1960: Architecture and Urbanism Between the Second World War and the Bicentennial* (Cologne: Taschen, 1997), 97; Guy Oakes, *The Imaginary War: Civil Defense and American Cold War Culture* (New York: Oxford University Press, 1994), 165.
6. On Du Bois, see: Chris Fuller, "Cora Du Bois and Twentieth-Century American Anthropology," *Anthropology of this Century*, http://aotcpress.com/articles/cora-du-bois-twentiethcentury-american-anthropology.

7   Carola Speads, *Breathing: The ABCs* (New York: Harper & Row, 1978). Republished twice as *Ways to Better Breathing* (Great Neck: Felix Morrow, 1986, and Rochester: Healing Arts Press, 1992).
8   Leo Kofler, *Die Kunst des Atmens: Als Grundlage der Tonerzeugung für Sänger, Schauspieler, Redner, Lehrer* (Kassel: Bärenreiter, 1986 [1897]).
9   Brett C. Millier, *Elizabeth Bishop: Life and the Memory of It* (Berkeley: University of California Press, 1993), 231–232; see also: Marilyn May Lombardi, "The Closet of Breath: Elizabeth Bishop, Her Body, and Her Art," *Twentieth-Century Literature* 38:2 (1992): 152–175. For contemporary artists see: Jean-Thomas Tremblay, *Breathing Aesthetics* (Durham: Duke University Press, 2022).
10 Tyler Anbinder, *City of Dreams: The 400-Year Epic History of Immigrant New York* (Boston: Houghton Mifflin, 2017), 500–503; Deborah Dwork and Robert Jan van Pelt, *Flight from the Reich: Refugee Jews, 1933–1946* (New York: Norton, 2012), 268–272; Michael Winkler, "Metropole New York," *Exilforschung* 20 (2002), 178–198.
11 Lori Gemeiner Bihler, *Cities of Refuge: German Jews in London and New York, 1935–1945* (Albany: SUNY Press, 2018), 112–114.
12 Hungry Gerald, "More Schlag, Please, Herr Doktor," *Hungry Gerald* (June 4, 2011), http://hungrygerald.com/2011/06/more-schlag-please-herr-doktor.
13 Allan M. Brandt, *The Cigarette Century: The Rise, Fall, and Deadly Persistence of the Product That Defined America* (New York: Basic Books, 2007), 99.
14 See Parker's column between 1942 and 1944, titled "Beauty" on Sundays and "The Beauty Quest" all other days of the week in *The New York Times*, https://timesmachine.nytimes.com.
15 Louis B. Schlivek, *Man in Metropolis: A Book about the People and Prospects of a Metropolitan Region* (New York: Doubleday, 1965), 167–169.
16 Paula A. Michaels, *Lamaze: An International History* (New York: Oxford University Press, 2014), 122; Marjorie Karmel, *Thank You, Dr. Lamaze: How One Mother Discovered the Deeply Satisfying Experience of Painless Childbirth* (New York: Dolphin, 1959).

17 On Lazarus and the context of her poem see Esther Schor, *Emma Lazarus* (New York: Schocken, 2006), 186–190.
18 For context: In London, England, in December 1952, thousands died in the worst fog the capital had ever seen. See Christine L. Corton, *London Fog: The Biography* (Cambridge: Belknap, 2015), 279–285.
19 Edith Evans Asbury, "Smog Is Really Smaze," *The New York Times* (November 21, 1953), 1; "How Do You Like Smog?" *The New York Times* (November 21, 1953), 12; "Smog, Smaze, Smoze, Smag," *The New York Times* (November 27, 1953), 26.

Wandervögel

1 Winfried Mogge, "Aufbruch einer Jugendbewegung: Wandervogel – Mythen und Fakten," *Fokus Wandervogel: Der Wandervogel in seinen Beziehungen zu den Reformbewegungen vor dem Ersten Weltkrieg*, ed. Sabine Weißler (Marburg: Jonas Verlag, 2001), 9–25.
2 Wedemeyer-Kolwe, *"Der neue Mensch:" Körperkultur im Kaiserreich und in der Weimarer Republik* (Würzburg: Königshausen & Neumann, 2004), 153–158, 178; Wedemeyer-Kolwe, *Aufbruch: Die Lebensreform in Deutschland* (Darmstadt: Philipp von Zabern, 2017), 32–35; Ulrich Linse, "Das 'natürliche' Leben: Die Lebensreform," *Erfindung des Menschen: Schöpfungsträume und Körperbilder 1500–2000*, ed. Richard van Dülmen (Vienna: Böhlau, 1998), 435–456.
3 Marion de Ras, *Körper, Eros und weibliche Kultur: Mädchen im Wandervogel und in der Bündischen Jugend 1900–1933* (Pfaffenweiler: Centaurus, 1988), 23.
4 Konrad Herter, *Begegnungen mit Menschen und Tieren: Erinnerungen eines Zoologen 1891–1978* (Berlin: Duncker & Humblot, 1979), 112.
5 Rainer Kramer, "Neuer Name: Margarete Draeger – Christin, Lehrerin, aufrechte Demokratin und Lebensretterin," *Gemeindereport Marienfelde* (September 2011), 12–13.
6 Bess M. Mensendieck, *Funktionelles Frauenturnen* (Munich: Bruckmann, 1930), 15.

7 Maren Möhring, *Marmorleiber: Körperbildung in der deutschen Nacktkultur* (Cologne: Böhlau, 2004), 64–68.
8 De Ras, *Körper, Eros und weibliche Kultur*, 168–169.
9 For Joachimson's (Jackson's) biography see: Helmut G. Asper, "Die unfreiwilligen Verwandlungen des Felix Joachimson," *Berlin, April 1933 by Felix Jackson* (Aachen: Alano, 1993), 265–296.
10 Wedemeyer-Kolwe, "Der neue Mensch," 25, 104–107.
11 Clara Schlaffhorst, "Die Bedeutung der Atmung," *Künstlerische Körperschulung*, ed. Ludwig Pallat and Franz Hilker (Breslau: Ferdinand Hirt, 1923), 71–80.
12 Katharina Scheel, *Modelle und Praxiskonzepte der Physiotherapie: Eine Verortung innerhalb von Anthropologie und Ethik* (Münster: Lit, 2013), 126.
13 Wedemeyer-Kolwe, "Der neue Mensch," 30; Hedwig Müller and Patricia Stöckemann, *"...jeder Mensch ist ein Tänzer:" Ausdruckstanz in Deutschland zwischen 1900 und 1945* (Gießen: Anabas, 1993), 31–41; Maggie Odom, "Mary Wigman: The Early Years, 1913–1925," *The Drama Review* 24:4 (1980), 81–92.
14 Werner E. Gerabek, "Lungentuberkulose," *Enzyklopädie Medizingeschichte*, ed. Werner E. Gerabek et al. (Berlin: De Gruyter, 2004) 871 ff.; Flurin Condrau, *Lungenheilanstalt und Patientenschicksal: Sozialgeschichte der Tuberkulose in Deutschland und England im späten 19. und frühen 20. Jahrhundert* (Göttingen: Vandenhoeck & Ruprecht, 2000), 276–281.
15 Sophie Ludwig, *Elsa Gindler–Von ihrem Leben und Wirken: "Wahrnehmen, was wir empfinden"* (Hamburg: Christians, 2002), 11–26.
16 Ludwig, 81.
17 Elsa Gindler, "Die Gymnastik des Berufsmenschen," *Elsa Gindler*, 83–93.
18 Sylvia Cserny, "Zur Entwicklung und Geschichte der KBT," *Der Körper ist der Ort des psychischen Geschehens: Grundlagenwissen der Konzentrativen Bewegungstherapie*, ed. Sylvia Cserny and Christa Paluselli (Würzburg: Königshausen & Neumann, 2006), 31–65.

19 Ruth C. Cohn, "Vorwort zur deutschen Ausgabe," *Atmen: Eine illustrierte Anleitung zur natürlichen Atmung* by Carola Speads (Munich: Kösel, 1983), 7–10.
20 See Theodolinda Aldenhoven on the introduction to a Gindler course taught as late as 1937 (*Erinnerungen an Elsa Gindler: Berichte, Briefe, Gespräche mit Schülern* [Munich: P. Zeitler, 2000], 105). All other details follow Gindler's course notes taken in the years 1927/28. See Edith von Arps-Aubert, *Das Arbeitskonzept von Elsa Gindler (1885–1961) dargestellt im Rahmen der Gymnastik der Reformpädagogik* (Hamburg: Kovac, 2010), 388–393.
21 Helen Boak, *Women in the Weimar Republic* (Manchester: Manchester University Press, 2013), 279; see also: Lynne Frame, "Gretchen, Girl, Garçonne? Weimar Science and Popular Culture in Search of the Ideal New Woman," *Women in the Metropolis: Gender and Modernity in Weimar Culture*, ed. Katharina von Ankum (Berkeley: University of California Press, 1997), 12–40.
22 Gindler, "Zur Gymnastik des Berufsmenschen," *Elsa Gindler*, 91.
23 Quoted in: Arps-Aubert, *Das Arbeitskonzept von Elsa Gindler*, 388–393.
24 Hans-Ulrich Thamer, *Alltag in Berlin: Das 20. Jahrhundert* (Berlin: Eisengold, 2016), 14.
25 On Weimar culture see Sabina Becker, *Experiment Weimar: Eine Kulturgeschichte Deutschlands 1918–1933* (Darmstadt: Wissenschaftliche Buchgesellschaft, 2018), 26–32, 219, 227; Ursula Büttner, *Weimar: Die überforderte Republik* (Stuttgart: Klett-Cotta, 2008), 333.
26 Ludwig, *Elsa Gindler*, 65.
27 Elke Mühlleitner, *Ich – Fenichel: Das Leben eines Psychoanalytikers im 20. Jahrhundert* (Vienna: Zsolnay, 2008), 146ff.
28 Otto Fenichel, *Psychoanalyse und Gymnastik*, ed. Johannes Reichmayr (Gießen: Psychosozial, 2015).
29 Otto Fenichel, "Über Respiratorische Introjektion," *Internationale Zeitschrift für Psychoanalyse* 17 (1931), 234–255.
30 Otto Fenichel, "The Psychopathology of Coughing," *Psychosomatic Medicine* 5 (1943), 181–184.
31 Gindler, "Zur Gymnastik des Berufsmenschen," 84.

Notice What Is

1. Saul Friedländer, *Nazi Germany and the Jews, Vol. I: The Years of Persecution, 1933–1939* (New York: HarperCollins, 1997), 139.
2. Stern/Mellins/ Fishman, *New York 1960*, 666.
3. Russell B. Olwell, *At Work in the Atomic City: A Labor and Social History of Oak Ridge, Tennessee* (Knoxville: University of Tennessee Press, 2004), 1–5.
4. Gregg Mitman, *Breathing Space: How Allergies Shape Our Lives and Landscape* (New Haven: Yale University Press, 2008), 141–152; Julie Sze, *Noxious New York: The Racial Politics of Urban Health and Environmental Justice* (Cambridge: MIT Press, 2006), 91–108.
5. A survey of the conference contributions can be found in a German journal dedicated to breathing therapy: *Atem und Mensch: Vierteljahreszeitschrift für Atempflege, Atemtherapie und Atempädagogik* 3 (1959); for Isbert's first career see: Otto-Albrecht Isbert, *Volksboden und Nachbarschaft der Deutschen in Europa* (Langensalza: Beltz, 1937). For van Heeckeren see Hans-Harald Niemeyer, "Mit achtzig aktiv für eine bessere Welt," *Freiburger Yoga-Schule* (May 1988), https://www.freiburger-yogaschule.de/robert-van-heeckeren.
6. Charlotte Selver, *Waking Up: The Work of Charlotte Selver*, ed. William C. Littlewood and Mary Alice Roche (Bloomington: Author House, 2004), 89–95.
7. Bryan Taylor, "How the Salad Oil Swindle of 1963 Nearly Crippled the NYSE," *Business Insider* (23 November 2013), https://www.businessinsider.com/the-great-salad-oil-scandal-of-1963-2013-11?IR=T; see also: Norman C. Miller, *The Great Salad Oil Swindle* (New York: Coward McCann, 1965).
8. Marion Goldman, *The American Soul Rush: Esalen and the Rise of Spiritual Privilege* (New York: New York University Press, 2012), 1–20; Jeffrey J. Kripal, *Esalen: America and the Religion of No Religion* (Chicago: University of Chicago Press, 2008).
9. Goldman, *The American Soul Rush*, 3ff.

10 Roy Rosenzweig and Elizabeth Blackmar, *The Park and the People: A History of Central Park* (Ithaca: Cornell University Press, 1998), 491–497.
11 *Freedom to Breathe: Report of the Mayor's Task Force on Air Pollution in the City of New York* (New York: Task Force, 1966), 9ff.
12 Robert W. Snyder, *Crossing Broadway: Washington Heights and the Promise of New York City* (Ithaca: Cornell University Press, 2014), 115–117; Stanley Corkin, *Starring New York: Filming the Grime and Glamour of the Long 1970s* (New York: Oxford University Press, 2011), 42ff.; Joanne Reitano, *The Restless City: A Short History of New York from Colonial Times to the Present* (New York: Routledge, 2010), 183; Brian Tochterman, *The Dying City: Postwar New York and the Ideology of Fear* (Chapel Hill: University of North Carolina Press, 2017), 1–12; Robert W. Snyder, "Crime," *Encyclopedia of New York City*, ed. Kenneth T. Jackson (New Haven: Yale University Press, 1995), 297–299.
13 Yosef Hayim Yerushalmi, *Haggadah and History* (Philadelphia: Jewish Publication Society, 2005), 13–14.
14 Christopher Lasch, *The Culture of Narcissism* (New York: Norton, 1991 [1979]), 42–48.
15 Lasch, 396.
16 Paul Vitello, "Peter Workman, Book Publisher with an Eye for Hits, Dies at 74," *The New York Times* (April 8, 2013), https://www.nytimes.com/2013/04/09/business/media/peter-workman-book-publisher-with-an-eye-for-hits-dies-at-74.html; see also: Robert Klara, "Why Modern Parents Are Still Reading *What to Expect When You're Expecting*,"*Adweek* (August 13, 2017), https://www.adweek.com/brand-marketing/why-modern-parents-are-still-reading-what-to-expect-when-youre-expecting.

The List of Jewish Gymnastics Instructors

1 Christoph Kreutzmüller, *Ausverkauf: Die Vernichtung der jüdischen Gewerbetätigkeit in Berlin 1930–1945* (Berlin: Metropol, 2012), 133–139.
2 Friedländer, *Nazi Germany and the Jews, Vol. I*, 12–13.

3 Wedemeyer-Kolwe, "Der neue Mensch," 393.
4 Erich Jantetz, "Der Aufmarsch," *Gymnastik und Volkstanz: Monatsschrift der Fachschaft Gymnastik im Reichsverband Deutscher Turn-, Sport- und Gymnastiklehrer* 12:1 (1937), 15ff.
5 Paula Diehl, "Körperbilder und Körperpraxen im Nationalsozialismus," *Körper im Nationalsozialismus: Bilder und Praxen*, ed. Paula Diehl (Paderborn: Wilhelm Fink/Ferdinand Schöningh, 2013), 9–30; see also: Hans-Ulrich Thamer, "Volksgemeinschaft: Mensch und Masse," *Erfindung des Menschen: Schöpfungsträume und Körperbilder 1500–2000*, ed. Richard van Dülmen (Vienna: Böhlau, 1998), 367–386.
6 Gabriela Wesp, *Frisch Fromm Fröhlich Frau: Frauen und Sport zur Zeit der Weimarer Republik* (Königstein: Helmer, 1998); Wedemeyer-Kolwe, "Der neue Mensch," 414–416.
7 Ludwig, *Elsa Gindler*, 46; Wedemeyer-Kolwe, "Der neue Mensch," 415.
8 Wedemeyer-Kolwe, "Der neue Mensch," 63–65.
9 Friedländer, *Nazi Germany and the Jews, Vol. I*, 137–138.
10 Jutta Klamt, *Vom Erleben zum Gestalten: Die Entfaltung schöpferischer Kräfte im Deutschen Menschen* (Berlin: Dorn, 1936); "Jutta Klamt," *Der Spiegel* (May 24, 1947), 13.
11 Florence Moehl, "Flora Türkel (geb. Deutsch)," *Stolpersteine in Berlin*, https://www.stolpersteine-berlin.de/de/biografie/7333.
12 August Glucker, *Frisch und frei! Gymnastik der Frau in allen Lebensaltern* (Stuttgart: Franckh, 1936), 3, 10–11.
13 Robert N. Proctor, *The Nazi War on Cancer* (Princeton: Princeton University Press, 1999), 173–247.
14 Julia Franke, *Paris – eine neue Heimat? Jüdische Emigranten aus Deutschland 1933–1939* (Berlin: Duncker & Humblot, 2000), 52. Wolfgang Benz points out how much more difficult and expensive emigrating from Germany became after 1935, in comparison to the first two years of Nazi rule. See: Benz, "Das Exil der kleinen Leute," *Das Exil der kleinen Leute: Alltagserfahrungen deutscher Juden in der Emigration*, ed. Wolfgang Benz (Frankfurt: Fischer, 1994), 9–45.
15 Hans Surén, *Atemgymnastik: Die Schule der Atmung für Körper und Geist für alle Leibesübungen und Berufe* (Stuttgart: Franckh, 1937). For

Surén's biography see: Dietger Pforte, "Hans Surén – eine deutsche FKK-Karriere," *"Wir sind nackt und nennen uns Du:" Von Lichtfreunden und Sonnenkämpfern. Eine Geschichte der Freikörperkultur*, ed. Michael Andritzky and Thomas Rautenberg (Gießen: Anabas, 1989), 130–145. For Nazi ideology and discourses on the body see Diehl, "Körperbilder und Körperpraxen im Nationalsozialismus" and also: Janosch Steuwer, *"Ein Drittes Reich, wie ich es auffasse:" Politik, Gesellschaft und privates Leben in Tagebüchern 1933–1939* (Göttingen: Wallstein, 2017), 279–281.

16 For Solms' biography see: Rebecca Schwoch, *Jüdische Ärzte als Krankenbehandler in Berlin zwischen 1938 und 1945* (Frankfurt: Mabuse, 2018), 522.

17 For Schnell's biography see: "About Alfred Schnell," *Joods Monument* (April 7, 2016), https://www.joodsmonument.nl/en/page/507885/about-alfred-schnell.

18 Franke, *Paris – eine neue Heimat?*, 344.

19 Franke 125.

20 Jochen Thies, *Evian 1938: Als die Welt die Juden verriet* (Essen: Klartext, 2017).

21 Richard Breitman and Alan M. Kraut, *American Refugee Policy and European Jewry, 1933–1945* (Bloomington: Indiana University Press, 1987), 73ff.; Valerie Popp, *"Aber hier war alles anders…:" Amerikabilder der deutschsprachigen Exilliteratur nach 1939 in den USA* (Würzburg: Königshausen & Neumann, 2008), 53–66.

22 Franke, *Paris – eine neue Heimat?*, 300ff.

23 Michael L. Grace, "Sailing aboard the SS Champlain," *Cruiseline History* (13 June 2018), https://www.cruiselinehistory.com/1930s-sailing-1k1/; Andrea Pitzer, "Nabokov's Wartime Escape on the SS Champlain," *The Secret History of Vladimir Nabokov* (April 4, 2013), http://nabokovsecrethistory.com/news/nabokov-escape-to-america-records-ss-champlain/#.XDXri81CdZV.

24 Steven M. Lowenstein, "The German-Jewish Community of Washington Heights," *American Jewish Life, 1920–1990*, ed. Jeffrey S. Gurock (New York: Routledge, 1998), 245–254.

25 Anton Zischka, *Brot für zwei Milliarden Menschen* (Leipzig: Wilhelm Goldmann, 1938), 339.
26 *Aufbau*, 28 November, 1941.

Flowers from Charlotte

1 Also born in Berlin, the young woman on the cover was the German American model Ellen Harth (later a prominent agent in the modeling business). As a model, Harth was famous for her avantgarde haircut, her eye make-up and her professionalism. See: "Ellen Harth, 71, Model and Agent," *Lulu's Couture* (October 27, 2009), http://www.luluscouture.com/lulus-fashion/ellen-harth-71-model-and-agent/.
2 The first German edition was titled *Atmen: Eine illustrierte Anleitung zur natürlichen Atmung* (Munich: Kösel, 1983). A 1987 edition was titled *Natürliches Atmen – intensiver und gesünder leben: Atemübungen helfen heilen* (Landsberg am Lech: mvg, 1987).
3 For a survey see: Steven Starker, *Oracle at the Supermarket: The American Preoccupation with Self-Help Books* (New Brunswick: Transaction, 2009).
4 Sheldon Saul Hendler, *The Oxygen Breakthrough: 30 Days to an Illness-Free Life* (New York: Pocket, 1989); Pam Grout, *Jumpstart Your Metabolism: How to Lose Weight by Changing the Way You Breathe* (New York: Simon & Schuster, 1998).
5 Jane Gross, "A New, Purified Form of Cocaine Causes Alarm as Abuse Increases," *The New York Times* (29 November 1985), 1; B 6; Howard Padwa and Jacob A. Cunningham, "Crack Epidemic," *Drugs in American Society: An Encyclopedia of History, Politics, Culture and the Law, Vol. I*, ed. Nancy E. Marion and Willard M. Oliver (Santa Barbara: ABC-CLIO, 2014), 228–230.
6 Anthony Storr, *Solitude* (London: Flamingo, 1990 [1988]), 12–15.
7 The poem opens "Part II" of Rilke's *Sonnets to Orpheus*: "Atmen, du unsichtbares Gedicht! / Immerfort um das eigne / Sein eingetauschter Weltraum. Gegengewicht, / in dem ich mich rhythmisch ereigne."

These lines and the English translation taken from: Rainer Maria Rilke, *The Sonnets to Orpheus*, translated by Leslie Norris and Alan Keele (Columbia: Camden House, 1989), 28.

8   *Reclaiming Vitality and Presence: Sensory Awareness as a Practice for Life*, ed. Richard Low and Stefan Laeng-Gilliatt (Berkeley: North Atlantic, 2007), 258–260.
9   Sze, *Noxious New York*, 91–108.
10 Mark Jackson, *Asthma: The Biography* (New York: Oxford University Press, 2009), 168–183, 203.
11 A 2012 study shows that three million deaths worldwide that year could be traced back to indoor or outdoor air pollution. See: World Health Organization, *Ambient Air Pollution: A Global Assessment of Exposure and Burden of Disease* (Geneva: WHO Press, 2016), 15; Beth Gardiner, *Choked: Life and Breath in the Age of Air Pollution* (Chicago: University of Chicago Press, 2019).
12 Carola H. Speads and Margaret J. Leong, "Breathing: An Approach for Facilitating Movement," *Therapeutic Considerations for the Elderly*, ed. Osa Littrup Jackson (London: Churchill Livingstone, 1987), 55–66.

Speads Work

1   Gabriel O. Apata, "'I Can't Breathe:' The Suffocating Nature of Racism," *Theory, Culture & Society* 37:7-8 (2020): 241–254; Omotayo T. Jolaosho, "The Enduring Urgency of Black Breath," *Anthropology News* (April 16, 2021), https://www.anthropology-news.org/articles/the-enduring-urgency-of-black-breath/.
2   Yale/New Haven Health/Bridgeport Hospital, "The Center for Sleep Medicine," https://www.bridgeporthospital.org/services/sleep-medicine.
3   Belisa Vranich, *Breathe: The Simple, Revolutionary 14-Day Program to Improve Your Mental and Physical Health* (New York: St Martin's Griffin, 2016); Dan Brulé, *Just Breathe: Mastering Breathwork* (New York: Atria, 2017).

4   Carl Gustav Jung, *Seelenprobleme der Gegenwart* (Olten: Walter, 1973 [1932]), 174–176.
5   For a survey and the expression "Ätherziege" ("ethereal she-goat") see: Karoline von Steinaecker, *Luftsprünge: Anfänge moderner Körpertherapien* (Munich: Urban & Fischer, 2000), 58.
6   Ernst Bloch, *Das Prinzip Hoffnung*, Vol. 2 (Frankfurt: Suhrkamp, 1973 [1959]), 542–545.
7   For a discussion of Gindler's work in an epistemological context see Katja Rothe, "The Gymnastics of Thought: Elsa Gindler's Networks of Knowledge," *Encounters of Performance Philosophy*, ed. Laura Cull and Alice Lagaay (London: Palgrave Macmillan, 2014), 197–219.
8   Jay Schleichkorn, *The Bobaths: A Biography of Bertha and Karel Bobath* (Tucson: Therapy Skill Builders, 1992), xi, 47; see also Berta Bobath's preface to Carola Speads, *Ways to Better Breathing* (Great Neck: William Morrow, 1986) n.pag.
9   On the impact of Gindler's work see: Judyth O. Weaver, "Der Einfluss von Elsa Gindler," *Handbuch der Körperpsychotherapie*, ed. Gustl Marlock and Halko Weiss (Stuttgart: Schattauer, 2006), 33–40.
10 Alois Prinz, *Hannah Arendt oder die Liebe zur Welt* (Berlin: Insel, 2012); Hertha Nathorff, *Das Tagebuch der Hertha Nathorff: Berlin-New York: Aufzeichnungen, 1933–1945* (Frankfurt: Fischer, 2016); for a case study of a gymnastics/bodywork expert who remained in Germany and survived in hiding, see: Mark Roseman, "Ein Mensch in Bewegung: Dore Jacobs (1894–1978)," *Essener Beiträge: Beiträge zur Geschichte von Stadt und Stift Essen* 114 (2002), 73–109.
11 Ronald E. Purser, *McMindfulness: How Mindfulness Became the New Capitalist Spirituality* (London: Repeater, 2019), 8–9; David Forbes, *Mindfulness and Its Discontents: Education, Self, and Social Transformation* (Nova Scotia: Fernwood, 2019).
12 "DOK. 146: Aaltje de Vries-Bouwes berichtet in ihrem Tagebuch am 29. Juni 1942 von Gerüchten, dass in Polen Hunderttausende von Juden vergast würden," *Die Verfolgung und Ermordung der europäischen Juden durch das nationalsozialistische Deutschland 1933–1945*, Vol. 5: *West- und Nordeuropa 1940-Juni 1942*, ed. Susanne Heim et al. (Munich: Oldenbourg, 2012), 399ff.

13 Anna Hájková, "Das Polizeiliche Durchgangslager Westerbork," *Terror im Westen: Nationalsozialistische Lager in den Niederlanden, Belgien und Luxemburg 1940–1945*, ed. Wolfgang Benz und Barbara Distel (Berlin: Metropol, 2004), 217–248.
14 Margaret S. Mahler, *Mein Leben, mein Werk*, ed. Paul E. Stepansky (Munich: Kösel, 1989), 127–131; Bernhard Handlbauer, "Wiener Psychoanalytikerinnen im US-amerikanischen Exil: Auswirkungen der Emigration auf berufliche Identität, Karriere und Lebenswerk," *Zwischenwelt 9: Frauen im Exil*, ed. Siglinde Bolbecher and Beate Schmeichel-Falkenberg (Klagenfurt: Drava, 2007), 201–223.
15 See for Schwarz's scholarship: *Die Wiedergutmachung nationalsozialistischen Unrechts durch die Bundesrepublik Deutschland, Vol. 1–7*, ed. Walter Schwarz (Munich: Beck, 1974–2000).
16 "Der Volkswagen: 75 Jahre VW Käfer," *Focus* (January 27, 2013), https://www.focus.de/auto/gebrauchtwagen/oldtimer/tid-29175/75-jahre-volkswagen-kaefer-vom-hitler-golf-zur-kult-kugel_aid_903982.html.
17 Achim Trunk, "Die todbringenden Gase," *Neue Studien zu nationalsozialistischen Massentötungen durch Giftgas: Historische Bedeutung, technische Entwicklung, revisionistische Leugnung*, ed. Günter Morsch and Bertrand Perz (Berlin: Metropol, 2011), 23–49; Astrid Ley, "Massentötung durch Kohlenmonoxid: Die 'Erfindung' einer Mordmethode, die 'Probevergasung' und der Krankenmord in Brandenburg/Havel," *Neue Studien zu nationalsozialistischen Massentötungen durch Giftgas*, 88–99.

Sources

1 On biography and its problematic aspects see: Hermione Lee, *Biography: A Very Short Introduction* (Oxford: Oxford University Press, 2009), 1–18.

Cultural Studies

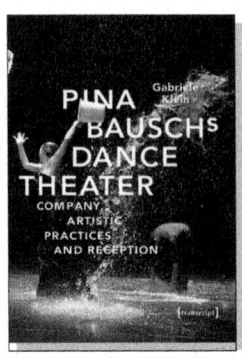

Gabriele Klein
Pina Bausch's Dance Theater
Company, Artistic Practices and Reception

2020, 440 p., pb., col. ill.
29,99 € (DE), 978-3-8376-5055-6
E-Book:
PDF: 29,99 € (DE), ISBN 978-3-8394-5055-0

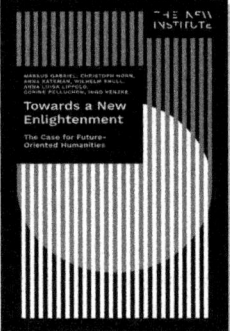

Markus Gabriel, Christoph Horn, Anna Katsman, Wilhelm Krull, Anna Luisa Lippold, Corine Pelluchon, Ingo Venzke
**Towards a New Enlightenment –
The Case for Future-Oriented Humanities**

October 2022, 80 p., pb.
18,00 € (DE), 978-3-8376-6570-3
E-Book: available as free open access publication
PDF: ISBN 978-3-8394-6570-7
ISBN 978-3-7328-6570-3

Sven Quadflieg, Klaus Neuburg, Simon Nestler (eds.)
(Dis)Obedience in Digital Societies
Perspectives on the Power of Algorithms and Data

March 2022, 380 p., pb., ill.
29,00 € (DE), 978-3-8376-5763-0
E-Book: available as free open access publication
PDF: ISBN 978-3-8394-5763-4
ISBN 978-3-7328-5763-0

**All print, e-book and open access versions of the titles in our list
are available in our online shop www.transcript-publishing.com**

Cultural Studies

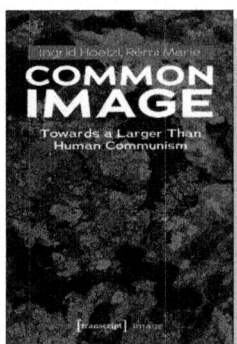

Ingrid Hoelzl, Rémi Marie
Common Image
Towards a Larger Than Human Communism

2021, 156 p., pb., ill.
29,50 € (DE), 978-3-8376-5939-9
E-Book:
PDF: 26,99 € (DE), ISBN 978-3-8394-5939-3

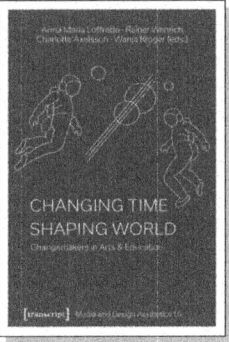

Anna Maria Loffredo, Rainer Wenrich,
Charlotte Axelsson, Wanja Kröger (eds.)
Changing Time – Shaping World
Changemakers in Arts & Education

September 2022, 310 p., pb., col. ill.
45,00 € (DE), 978-3-8376-6135-4
E-Book: available as free open access publication
PDF: ISBN 978-3-8394-6135-8

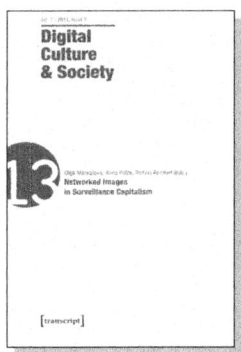

Olga Moskatova, Anna Polze, Ramón Reichert (eds.)
Digital Culture & Society (DCS)
Vol. 7, Issue 2/2021 –
Networked Images in Surveillance Capitalism

August 2022, 336 p., pb., col. ill.
29,99 € (DE), 978-3-8376-5388-5
E-Book:
PDF: 27,99 € (DE), ISBN 978-3-8394-5388-9

**All print, e-book and open access versions of the titles in our list
are available in our online shop www.transcript-publishing.com**